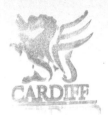
stop
smoking
87% success rate

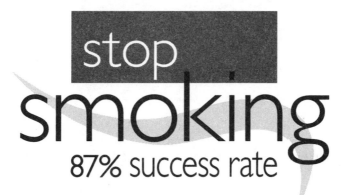

stop
smoking
87% success rate

it's all in your mind
and you can beat it

gillian bridge

foulsham
LONDON • NEW YORK • TORONTO • SYDNEY

foulsham

The Publishing House, Bennetts Close, Cippenham, Slough,
Berkshire, SL1 5AP, England

ISBN 0-572-03119-X

Cover photograph from Powerstock

A CIP record for this book is available from the British Library

Neither the editors of W. Foulsham & Co. Ltd nor the
author nor the publisher take responsibility for any
possible consequences from any treatment, procedure,
test, exercise, action or application of medication or
preparation by any person reading or following the
information in this book. The publication of this book
does not constitute the practice of medicine, and this
book does not attempt to replace any diet or
instructions from your doctor. The author and publisher
advise the reader to check with a doctor before
administering any medication or undertaking any
course of treatment or exercise.

Printed in Great Britain by Creative Print and Design (Wales), Ebbw Vale

Contents

Introduction

Or, Be Prepared

You've given up a lot of your life and your time to smoking cigarettes so now, as you prepare to stop smoking, you need to think about setting aside some time so that you can give stopping smoking the place in your life it deserves.

I'm not going to tell you it will be easy, but you can do it and I'm going to be with you all the way to help you. I've done it, and I've helped hundreds of others do it as well.

When we start to look at the practical aspects of giving up smoking, I'll give you plenty of reasons why you should think very seriously about taking a short holiday when you are stopping smoking – a weekend at least, or perhaps longer. It will help you to take a break from your normal routines so you can also break out of some of the old associations between cigarettes and your daily life. And, perhaps most importantly of all, when you're away from normal distractions you will be able to concentrate that much better on reading this book. You'll have the time to think about all the issues it's bound to raise for you, and carry out all the little tasks you'll find set out for you in these pages.

My system for helping you give up includes practical tasks – some even involving paper, scissors, felt tips, scraps of this and that and some sticky-backed plastic! This may sound odd but don't be put off because there are excellent reasons for doing them, and if you can let yourself go and really get into them, you'll have a lot of fun – and the great satisfaction of stirring up the curiosity of everyone around you!

So be prepared to give up a few days while you are reading this book. Give yourself all the time you can to stop smoking.

If you want to give up, with my help you can give up. And I'm going to be with you every step of the way. Good luck!

Quit While You're Ahead

Or, Stop smoking before your body stops for ever

Don't start reading this book unless you're absolutely certain you want to stop smoking – because it's going to work to change your life.

This book is revolutionary. It's going to be all about you and smoking, not about smoking and you. 'Smoking' can't be changed by reading a book – but you can! So if you're up for change, read this book carefully all the way to the end and you'll find that you and your life, finances and relationships will be changed for good – if that's what you really want.

Smoking can never be affected by a book or, in fact, by anything at all, because, despite all those images you see conjured up in posters and government warnings, smoking isn't a 'thing'. It isn't a monster, it isn't a dark force lurking 'out there', silently waiting to pounce on you and force you into a lifetime of slavery. Images of that kind don't help you to see your smoking in perspective. Instead they only reinforce the sense you may already have that you've lost control and are now a victim to cigarettes. You don't need that. The uncomfortable, but encouraging, reality is that the only force involved in what you do when you smoke is you. *You* are the 'thing' that makes smoking happen and without *you* … well, you can work out the rest!

That's all sad but true. But the fantastic upside is that it means that you can be in control of your own quitting process. And that's very good news.

Furthermore, you're not going to give up smoking: you're going to divide and conquer. Smoking is no more a single activity than it is a monster. From here on in, think of it instead as a toxic jumble of addictive thinking, fantasy images, ritual actions you carry out with little white tubes, and anxiety-producing, addictive, chemical effects. Ridding yourself of all these should be a positive pleasure.

Come on a journey with me to the end of this book and you will learn how to successfully challenge, change or overcome these elements of the artwork formerly known as 'smoking'. Discover how to separate and manage them. Learn to do what I have done for myself, and have helped many others to do – make cigarettes irrelevant to your life.

How sexy is a schlime?

Let's start the challenge with the very language of smoking. It comes complete with a certain chic romanticism attached to it: dark smoky eyes; elegant 1930s film stars with long cigarette holders; all that jazz. But let's try changing the language for a minute. Imagine a sultry Marlene Dietrich temptress shoving something called a 'schlime' between her lips, then 'muking' it to draw the (same old) toxins into her lungs. How chic or romantic does that sound? 'Oh, dahling, I'm simply gasping for a schlime!' How rock-hard can boys be if they're caught muking behind the bike sheds?

Why do you smoke?

Which begs the question, if there's really nothing intrinsically chic, romantic, sensible or, indeed, inescapable and involuntary involved in smoking, why on earth do you want to do it? Have you ever asked yourself the straight question: 'Why me?'

What is there about you, in particular, that you should have ended up wanting to do this rather strange and utterly harmful thing?

Read on if you're brave enough. Because you're going to find out.

You are unique. There's nobody else quite like you. Sure, there are lots of people out there who do similar things to you – but they will do them for different reasons. So, though lots and lots of people smoke, nobody else will smoke for quite the same reasons you do.

- You have your own very personal reasons for smoking.

- You have to have your own very personal reasons to stop smoking.

- And you have to have your very own personalised props to help you.

Which is why this book is different. It is arranged to help you. Nobody else. Just you.

How do others see you?

We can learn a lot about ourselves by first looking at other people. We've all said about someone else: 'They're their own worst enemy', at the same time thinking how easy it is to see straight through them to the cause of their self-destructive behaviour. We all like to indulge in a little analysis of those around us:

'He's at least twice her age, it'll all end in tears! Her trouble is that she's always looking for a father figure.'

'Third driving offence in six months – he's always thought himself above the law. That's what comes of being a spoilt only child.'

'How can she say she's on a diet when she's eating that – it must be a zillion calories. But what'll she hang her problems on if she does finally lose weight?'

And many of us are familiar with Robert Burns's (probably heartfelt) plea in *To a Louse*.

> *O wad some Pow'r the giftie gie us*
> *To see oursels as others see us!*
> *It wad frae mony a blunder free us,*
> *And foolish notion.*

We have to (reluctantly) acknowledge that we might save ourselves a lot of problems if only we would view our lives a bit more from the outside in, and less from the inside out! For the 'blunders and foolish notions' Burns mentions, read 'smoking and self-deceptions': by which I mean those sorry excuses that we've all come up with in the past, that have enabled us to carry on with our smoking behaviour. The time has come to be your own 'Power', to give yourself that 'giftie', and to be brave enough, with the support of this book, to see yourself as others might see you. This is the first step towards freeing yourself from all those excuses and the 'blunder' that your unwanted smoking behaviour has been up to now.

So, in the first place, how do other people see smokers in general?

Certainly not in the way that some smokers fondly seem to see themselves. Some (not you, I'm sure) seem drawn to an enticing fantasy that smoking is the automatic accessory of some rather sexy and fascinating lifestyles; that 'creative' people smoke; that 'driven' people smoke; that feisty, radical types smoke; that the people who are having the most fun smoke.

But what is the sad, day-to-day reality that more usually hits non-smokers between the eyes (and in the nose)?

Well, apart from the whiffy huddles of chilly smokers around the doors of office blocks and hospitals, and the mess of fag-ends on the ground, what they actually most often see when they're looking at smokers is:

- Eyes screwing up as smoke rises into them

- Lips puckering up as they suck greedily on an odd, white tube

- Wisps of smoke escaping from noses and mouths with every word that's spoken

- Fingers endlessly tap-tapping fag-ash off

- And a blind facility for ignoring the senses of people all around them in the self-absorbed pursuit of the sucking and the blowing and the tapping.

How genuinely fascinating, sophisticated, fun or sexy is that?

What about the even sadder reality that most alcoholics and virtually all schizophrenics and drug addicts, and millions of unemployed and tragic people on every margin of society smoke, too. Picture all those teenage mothers pushing underweight babies in ash-covered pushchairs. How sophisticated and sexy is the reality now?

So, having called into question a few common delusions about smokers as a group, to follow up Robert Burns's point, the first big question we have to ask ourselves as individuals is:

'Seen from the outside in, how does my behaviour really look?'

Then we can move on to:

'Is it glaringly obvious to other people *why* I carry on with this behaviour?'

(And this is especially important if it's not a behaviour that we want to carry on with.)

Defensiveness

At this point you might be starting to feel a bit defensive, and that would be perfectly natural. But if so, what do you suppose you are feeling defensive about? The smoking itself? No, you already know smoking is hard to defend. You know that nothing else in your personal life, apart from alcohol, drugs, mental illness or body odour, does so much to harm your health, wealth, relationships, freedom, fertility, sexiness, good looks, clothes – and your future. If you didn't recognise all that you wouldn't be reading this book. No, it's not smoking you're defending.

What you might instinctively feel defensive about, though, is who you are. It's something we all share, and want to protect. And you're probably getting the idea (quite rightly) that this book is going to say that you'll have to adjust your sense of who you are. That quitting smoking is going to involve more than changing a single mode of behaviour: it's going to mean partly changing who you are at the moment. The bonus is that, like all of us who have successfully quit, you will feel much more comfortable with who you go on to become. As well as being extraordinarily proud of what you have achieved as a result.

Smoking as a smokescreen

Anyone can give up smoking for a while – you've possibly already done it yourself. But smoking is literally a smokescreen: it covers up something else, and unless that something else is dealt with at the same time as the smoking behaviour, it won't simply go away. In fact, once the smoking behaviour is removed, whatever lies behind it may stand out even more and will certainly be the cause of any future relapses.

So what sort of thing is smoking a smokescreen for? Well, smoking is like most other addictive behaviours in that although smoking addiction turns into a physical thing – the body becomes chemically dependent on nicotine – the addiction doesn't start out as a physical need. It's all in the mind. After all, nobody has to have that first cigarette; it is not a physical necessity in the way that food and drink are. Smoking starts because of something in the way we think. Or, to put it another way, it's mental. (In all senses!)

If that seems difficult to believe, simply ask yourself why, if smoking is purely a physical addiction (which is the accepted wisdom behind some treatments), so many people go back to smoking, having previously given it up for months or even years? After all, the nicotine has long since left the body; within a relatively short period of time there won't be a trace of chemical dependency involved. The tricky reality – the one that this book uniquely is going to deal with – is that the only dependency left is the mental one.

This is why, if you really want to quit smoking for good, you need more help than chemical help. The effect of chemical treatment for addiction can only last so long. And you don't want to complicate the issue by risking replacing one form of chemical dependency with another, when working on the root cause of your smoking – the way in which you think – will bring really effective and longer-lasting results.

Defensiveness, though natural, is only going to get in the way of the process. If you do feel it, just ride with it for now. Think about what you are aiming to achieve and how much you want to achieve it.

Ambivalence

The other potential barrier to getting the most out of this book is that you may not, even at this stage, be absolutely sure that you *do* want to quit smoking. Lots of us have felt that way, even when we've told the world we're about to quit. You probably expected and recognise this ambivalence, but you need to understand that there is a hidden reason for what you're feeling. Quitting cigarettes has the impact of a mini-bereavement. You're going to be saying goodbye to your one firm, loyal and uncritical friend, the one who's been there for you when all else has failed, when all the world's been against you. So, although you know the deed's got to be done, when it comes down to the wire you may still find yourself coming up with lots of objections to what you're reading and about to read. Ignore them. Put on a black armband for now and bear with them: you may be sure that by the end of the book not only will you be glad you've stuck with it, but you'll also be raring to party in rainbow colours.

It may also help to know that there could actually be a physiological basis for the ambivalence that you almost certainly feel. It may be a result of the two-sided way our brains work. The two halves of the brain are linked by a connecting structure called the *corpus callosum*. If it gets damaged and the two halves can't work together any more, our hands (each linked to one half of the brain) may start behaving independently. One unhappy smoker who'd suffered corpus callosum damage was driven demented as her left hand kept throwing away cigarettes as her right hand was trying to light them! The intuitive right half of her brain (probably recognising how harmful smoking is to the body) was telling its connected hand to do its damnedest to stop her smoking. Apparently, she was quite literally in two minds about what she wanted to do!

So, if you *are* feeling in two minds right now, keep reminding yourself that you won't be in two minds about the benefits of quitting once you've achieved all that guilt-free good health. Let your intuitive brain dominate – you know it's right!

How you think about smoking

Whatever you're feeling, it's what we *think* about our feelings that drives what we do. Even hardened smokers don't absolutely have to light up every time they feel like it, they can think themselves out of it. There aren't many people who would automatically light up in front of the Queen. You probably spend more of your life not smoking than smoking, so what is it about those times when you do light up that sets them apart? What are your thought processes doing then?

And that is where we came in: you've got to look at your thinking. Soon, very soon, there will come that exciting stage in the book when you're going to work out all the things that have affected and still affect the way you think; the ones that outsiders might currently find easier to spot than you do, and which have resulted in your smoking behaviour. First, though, you need to be able to see that behaviour for what it is. So the next stage is to do that Robert Burns thing and 'see yourself as others see you'. This will help you in two ways:

1   By killing the idea of the 'smoking monster'. When you look at yourself more objectively, you will see a simple set of behaviours you're going to change.

2   By taking ownership and recognising you're in charge. These are *your* specific and individual behaviours so they are *yours* to control and change.

The time has come to look at what you're going to stop doing. In the next chapter, we are going to examine what it is that you actually do when you smoke.

Mirror, Mirror on the Wall

Or, Take a long, hard look at yourself

We're now going to take a close look at what you are actually doing when you smoke – to see yourself as others see you. The questions are designed to help you work out what your smoking behaviour really consists of and looks like. Write your answers down as you go. This will help you focus on what you're doing and prevent your mind from wandering. Also, you'll be needing those answers again later.

Your smoking behaviour

1   When do you light up a cigarette?

    a   At set times of the day, i.e., to a regular pattern, such as with meals, at coffee breaks, etc. ☐

    b   Occasionally, i.e., when prompted by particular occasions, such as experiencing strong feelings (e.g. nervousness) or events (e.g. a trip to the pub), rather than according to pre-set patterns ☐

    c   All the time, that is, you chain-smoke ☐

2   How many cigarettes do you buy per week? ⬚

3   How many cigarettes do you actually put in your mouth per week? (Include those given to you as well as those bought by you.) ⬚

4   Do you mostly smoke cigarettes:

    a   Alongside other consumables, such as food, drink, drugs? ☐

    b   By themselves? ☐

    If (a), would cigarettes taste different if consumed by themselves? Yes/No

5   Do you mostly stand or sit
    when having a cigarette?   ☐

6   Do you mostly smoke cigarettes:

    a   Indoors (including in cars)?   ☐

    b   Out of doors?   ☐

    c   Both?   ☐

7   Do you smoke cigarettes while:

    a   Standing still in one place?   ☐

    b   Moving around?   ☐

8   Do you smoke cigarettes when working?   Yes/No

9   Do you smoke cigarettes when relaxing?   Yes/No

10 In what company do you usually smoke cigarettes?

    a   Your own   ☐

    b   Mostly with other people   ☐

    c   Mostly with other smokers   ☐

11 Do you have a cigarette when you don't want to think?   Yes/No

12 Do you have a cigarette when you want to think more
    clearly?   Yes/No

13 Do you organise and budget for your cigarette buying?   Yes/No

14 Do you buy cigarettes on impulse?   Yes/No

15 Are cigarettes part of your everyday shopping?   Yes/No

16 Do you buy cigarettes with other 'leisure time' goods,
    e.g. wine, magazines, etc.?   Yes/No

17 Is going out to buy cigarettes an important activity?   Yes/No

Ceremonials

You will almost certainly have a number of rituals – we'll call them 'ceremonials' that you adhere to (consciously or otherwise) when you smoke. These are to do with the way you take cigarettes out of their packet, light them, hold them, dispose of them, and so on.

1   Do you open cigarette packets carefully, or rip them open?

2   What do you do with the silver foil?

3   Do you throw rubbish carefully into containers or chuck it down anywhere?

4   How do you release a cigarette from the pack: do you tap it or pull it out?

5   Do you close the pack lid or leave it open?

6   When you light the cigarette, do you use a lighter or matches?

7   Does it matter which?   Yes/No

8   Do you have a special lighter?   Yes/No

9   Does it feel wrong if you change your method?   Yes/No

10 When you light a cigarette, do you grip it between your lips or hold it in place by hand?

11 Write down all the details of how you hold the cigarette, inhale and generally physically behave during the time you are actually using the cigarette as a source of smoke. For example: Do you keep the cigarette in your mouth more often than not? Do you flick ash constantly or tap a long section of it on to a container? Do you draw smoke into your lungs right to the end or only at the start? Add any others that occur to you.

12 Do you consume the cigarette quickly or slowly?

13 Do you consume a cigarette right down to the butt?

14 How do you extinguish a cigarette: in a formal place or anywhere, on the ground, in a cup, etc.?

15 How do you dispose of a cigarette butt?

Assessing your smoking behaviour

The answers you gave to those questions may not have seemed very significant to you. Or it's possible that this was the first time you'd thought about and come face to face with smoking as a piece of real-time behaviour. Because that's just what it is: smoking is just something else you do, just another series of actions, like putting on your clothes or driving a car. And, as such, smoking is something that you have the capacity to control or alter.

Looking at your smoking behaviour should help you to understand that smoking is not some absurdly romanticised power that you have to give in to. If you can see quitting in terms of ending a series of rather dreary activities, rather than in terms of fighting off an evil but compulsively fulfilling thing that happens to be called smoking, you'll make it much easier on yourself, and make it pretty near certain you'll succeed.

Be objective

Now, let's use Robert Burns's magic formula again. Imagine that the answers you've just given were written up as a detailed description in a book and applied to a fictional character's smoking habits. What would you think about that person's smoking behaviour?

Taking the suggestion even further, how would you picture them and how would you judge or analyse their behaviour? Remembering how easy it is to sort out other people's problems (assuming you would see that smoking behaviour as a problem!), what advice could you imagine you would want to give to that person?

Take Matt as an example. There he is, happily smoking away whilst chatting to a gorgeous woman and remaining oblivious to how his smoking is affecting her (as well as his chances of 'scoring'). Think how he might gain the insight to change his behaviour if he was able to describe it to himself in the following way.

> *Matt inhaled deeply from his cigarette before turning towards the lovely Samantha. He moved ever closer to her as he fed her tales of his courageous exploits. But however compelling these might have been, she couldn't concentrate on them because all she was able to focus on was her own disgust at the wreaths of foul-smelling blue smoke she was encased in whenever his mouth opened to tell his story. She kept moving backwards, but still she couldn't quite escape the smoke and the*

accompanying spittle. Even the yellowing fingers that flicked ash indiscriminately over the ashtray and her skirt told a louder tale than his words. She didn't quite believe that such a man, despite his startling blue eyes, was the hero he described. She made her excuses and left.

Give it a go yourself. It really will pay off.

What do you get out of smoking?

By now you should have been able to identify a large part of your smoking behaviour, but unless you're way ahead of me, you won't have given any thought to what rewards you feel you are getting from it.

It would be very unnatural to choose to damage your health – which we all know you are doing – unless you felt you were getting some emotional benefit in return. I say 'emotional', since, as cigarettes basically fulfil no real physical need, the benefits or rewards must be in your head. No two heads being identical, the next task for you is to work out what your particular emotional rewards feel like, or mean, for you.

Think about the reward that you feel you are getting from that long process of buying a cardboard container of cigarettes, opening it, extracting one toxic tube, putting it between your lips, setting light to it, drawing the smoke into your lungs, playing finger puppets with it, using it as an aid to gesticulation, flicking ash from it, and crumpling the stub of it into a dirty ashtray. Not forgetting, of course, that whilst you're carrying out this lengthy business you're using up a lot of life that could be giving you other, more realistic, healthy and satisfactory kinds of reward.

Look at the following list of emotional 'rewards' and mark any that you feel apply to you.

I feel calmer. ☐

I feel life is more bearable. ☐

I feel less lonely; that I've got a friend. ☐

I feel I'm being defiant – and to hell with it. ☐

I feel I'm allowed to be angry. ☐

I feel sexy. ☐

I feel grown up. ☐

I feel macho. ☐

I feel less anxious. ☐

I feel soothed. ☐

I feel I've got 'time out'. ☐

I feel I belong. ☐

I feel less fat. ☐

I feel I can concentrate. ☐

I feel this is one of my few pleasures in life. ☐

I feel – I'm enjoying my fag. ☐

I feel – well, it's just a smoke, isn't it? ☐

Now write down any additional ones that apply to you that are not on the list.

Did you have to add any that weren't on the list? If you did, are you absolutely sure that they don't, in some way, fit into one of the categories above? And hopefully if you added to the list, you weren't tempted to make any sweeping claims that you really can't prove like, 'They make me sexier'!

Your earliest smoking behaviour

There is only one more small part of the picture of your smoking life that you need to look at now, after which we will start to work out how the person behind the smoking behaviour came about.

The last part of your smoking story is really the first part – where and when it all started. You probably don't actually remember your very first cigarette, as it may be lost behind the smokescreen of time, but if you have a very good memory and can remember it, concentrate on that particular one as you answer the following questions. If, like most of us, you don't remember a specific occasion and cigarette, just draw on your closest memories, but be as honest as possible about them. And keep on writing your answers down.

1 How old were you when you first put a lighted cigarette to your lips?

2 What was the background to you having that first cigarette? What was going on in your life at the time?

3 Describe your whereabouts when you had your first cigarette, that is, your physical position: were you sitting comfortably, standing, crouching whilst hiding, etc.?

4 If you were a child, where were your parents? Did they know?

5 Who bought the packet of cigarettes?

6   Did you *want* to try one or did you try it because you would have been made to feel bad if you hadn't (i.e., peer pressure)?

7   What was the sensation of holding the cigarette?

8   What was the sensation of drawing in the smoke?

9   Afterwards how did you feel about

   a   The cigarette?

   b   Yourself?

10 Did you mean to carry on with the smoking behaviour?

11 Picture the scene you remember as if you were watching someone else, not yourself, doing those things: as if you saw, not 'me' lighting that first fag (of how many?), but simply a small child, an anxious adult, whatever stage you happened to be at when you had that first cigarette. How would you react now if you could see it all happening in front of your eyes?

12 What would you want to do?

13 Would you want to try to prevent that (small? young?)
person from having that first cigarette?   Yes/No

14 Would you want to reach out and take care of them?   Yes/No

15 Would you want to counteract the influence of whatever it
was that had led to them wanting to try it in the first place?

Giving up

You've now looked at some of the history of your smoking behaviour
and should be realising that it isn't a dark monster after all, but when
broken down is simply a series of actions, from which you feel you get a
series of rewards. You've also tried to stand outside yourself a bit more
than usual, so you should have a better idea of what your smoking
behaviour looks like to the outside world and, Heaven knows, that might
be enough to put you off cigarettes already! But, sadly, probably not for
ever. Everyone knows how easy it can be to give up cigarettes. As Mark
Twain said, 'I can quit smoking if I wish: I've done it a thousand times.'

The reality is that to quit *for good* you need to do three things:

1 You need to get to the bottom of why you started in the first place.

2 You need to discover what primitive 'need' (in addition to the
immediate nicotine rush) gets rewarded every time you perform that
repetitive series of actions, as well as what current circumstances still
trigger that primitive need.

3 You need to challenge the needy feeling and find new ways to think
about it and manage it, so that the old, familiar series of smoking
actions becomes completely irrelevant to you.

That's the only certain way of preventing a relapse. And with the advice
and support of this book, doing those things is going to be relatively
simple and painless. In fact you've started on them already, and it hasn't
hurt so far, has it?

So hang on to your hat. Things are going to speed up now; you're
on your way to that bright new future.

The Big Birds of Influence

Or, How you developed addictive tendencies

As I've said before, it is ever so easy to see into the root causes of other people's behaviour; to see how their personalities were formed and to work out why they do the things they do. It can seem even easier to see through the excuses they make for their smoking behaviour: 'It's such a stressful job'; 'All my friends smoke'; 'I only have the occasional one when I'm given it'. To which we've probably all thought, 'Yeah, right!'

And that's why this book is encouraging you to see yourself a bit more from the outside in, as if you were someone else. It will make it easier to consider the causes of your own unwanted behaviour in as objective a light as possible, so that you will also find it easier to be tough on the excuses you've been giving yourself over the years for this behaviour.

You need to keep up that objectivity and gutsiness through the following section, because you're going to look at some very personal stuff now: the history of the formation of your own personality and the root causes of that particular unwanted behaviour – smoking. You're going to uncover the origins of that neediness (which we talked about at the end of the last chapter), which can only be satisfied by those strange things called cigarettes.

Later on, you will put what you discover here into a package, together with the answers you gave to those questions in the previous chapter. And when you put the two together you will see that, in day-to-day situations, you smoke in response to particular triggers – at certain times, in certain places, or in certain circumstances. In other words, when that neediness from the past is strongest.

Then, once you can recognise both the underlying needy feeling and the circumstances and occasions that are likely to stimulate or aggravate it, bingo, you have identified the ingredients of what I'm going to call the 'trigger moment'. That's the moment that usually results in you reaching for a pack of cigarettes. If you can learn to recognise a trigger moment for what it is, you will be able to defy any such moments (and all the old baggage they carry) *before* they can tempt you into any more harmful behaviour.

You will also see that, in the past, you've been as addicted to all those old behaviours as you have to the nicotine rushes themselves. We can then challenge your need for those behaviours and help you to work out alternative, healthier and much more satisfying behaviours and ways of supplying your needs. Doing all these things will make smoking seem unnecessary and unpleasant – for good.

So, let's go back to your very beginning – a very good place to start!

Innocent beginnings

There you are, newborn, pink and fresh, with not a bad habit in sight. But, sadly, between now and whenever it is that the answer in your questionnaire says you put that first cigarette between your lips, all that is going to change. Something in your life will affect you so that continually deciding to keep putting cigarettes in your mouth becomes possible. For some other people, something in their lives will affect them so that making those decisions is *not* possible. Whatever that 'something' is, it is obviously vitally important. You're going to track down the 'something' in your life that triggered (and still triggers) your smoking behaviour. And you really do need to ferret out what it is, so that in the future you will always be able to recognise it, challenge it, and take action against it. This way lies quitting for good.

But first, let's move slightly further back to the time before you turned pink, to the very first seconds of existence – when you were just about to become part of the big wide world. What's the first thing you did? You took a breath: the breath of life. Only once your lungs started to work independently could you be transported into the world of sensations that is human life. Clean and pure, your lungs expanded for the first time to take in that gigantic, dizzying breath that turned you into a person, an oxygen-dependent, breathing, thinking human being, one who would go on to have a life as varied and colourful as yours has been. The rest of your life depended on that first big, beautiful breath making its way into those beautiful, pink, healthy, innocent lungs.

What an amazing moment that was! But whatever went wrong after that? Can you seriously imagine *wanting* to put a cigarette between those tiny lips or *intending* to pollute those perfect lungs?

Of course not! But something did go wrong. You *did* put a fag between those lips, you *are* polluting those lungs, you *did* make those choices and now you need to work out why. You're going to find out what the 'something' was that came between the perfection of that first breath and now. And after that you're going to start putting things right again.

First impressions of life

Let's give that 'something' a shape. Imagine that the first things you saw and heard after being born were birds: great big birds that were hovering above your head. Imagine that they stayed with you, always hovering overhead, right through your growing-up years, constantly dropping little bits of this and that (sometimes poo, sometimes pretty, glittery feathers) down on to you. No matter what else was happening in your life you could still see and hear them, even though you became so used to them you never really noticed that they were there.

How much of an impact do you think they and their 'droppings' would have had on your development? How much unconscious influence do you think they would have had on the way you experienced things, including the way you thought about yourself and about life?

Well, childhood isn't usually dominated by big birds and their droppings (leaving aside Alfred Hitchcock), but it is dominated by influences, which, even though we may take them for granted, condition how we see and hear things, and dump their attitudes, their expectations, and their comments on us. Childhood is filled with people and experiences that influence us hugely and which, like big birds, get between us and everything else in the sky. They affect the look and the sound of everything around us when we are young, and their 'droppings', to a greater or lesser extent, still stick with us even as the very grown-up people we are today.

The 'something', then, that gets between the first breath and now, and which results in our smoking, is made up of two parts:

- The sense of self we develop as a response to the presence of 'birds' in our lives

- The beliefs we hold about life and our part in it, which developed as a result of the 'droppings', or messages, that landed on us.

It all started when we were *very* young. We were affected by the ways we were looked at, spoken to and handled from birth itself onwards.

From Day One we developed ways of feeling about ourselves (and very simple ways of thinking about ourselves) as a direct result of the way we were treated. Basically, this formed a simple self-image and, in a circular way, our self-image, and then went on to affect both the way we feel about present issues and (as a result of that) our behaviours themselves.

How the birds impacted on your self image

Did those around you look at you and respond to you empathetically when you were small, or were they often busy, tired, or 'not available'? Did your carers react calmly to your cries when you were hungry, thirsty or uncomfortable, or were their reactions irritable, nervous or agitated?

Needless to say, you won't actually remember how you were dealt with then, at least not consciously – but an inner part of you will remember and as a result will carry an image of who you are, how you should feel, and what responses are the norm for your life. So, even now, as the cool, young urban professional, macho leader of men, or grumpy old barfly that you are, you will still respond to daily issues in ways that were shaped by your earliest experience. And it will probably come as no surprise to you that the style of your response will ultimately be involved in whether or not you smoke.

Styles of coping

We all have different ways of coping with life's issues. Your answers to the following questions will help to establish your individual methods. In each case, tick the answer that applies to you. Write down any comments you may have on extra paper.

Control

Do you feel a need to be in charge all the time, in case you'll suffer in some way if you're not? ☐

Or, do you go with the flow? ☐

Gratification

When you feel hungry, thirsty or desire something badly, do you feel you should have what you want straight away, and feel worked up inside if you can't? ☐

Or, do you take time to think about your needs and perhaps choose to wait a bit to get the best or most sensible option? ☐

Frustration

If you can't have what you want, or something you're
doing isn't working out, do you get badly rattled? ☐

Or, do you turn your attention to something different or
look for a new way of tackling the thing? ☐

Anger

Do you control your anger? ☐

Or, does it control you? ☐

Hurt

When you feel hurt (physically or emotionally) do
you feel a stronger impulse to soothe your hurt and
make yourself feel better? ☐

Or, do you lash out at the cause of it or at something
else nearby? ☐

Impatience

Do you want everything now? ☐

Or, can you wait quietly as situations evolve? ☐

Selfishness

Do you secretly feel you should have the last slice of cake? ☐

Or, do you feel more comfortable sharing it? ☐

Anxiety

Does a generalised fear of losing everything, of everything
going 'belly-up', or of not being able to cope get in the way
of your being able to work things out or deal with life? ☐

Or, do you put life into context and take heart from looking
at the bigger picture? ☐

Interpreting your answers

The responses you gave there will give a very strong indication of how you learnt to feel about yourself as a result of how you were dealt with when you were tiny. Just to illustrate the point: if as a tot you were handled nervously, looked at through frightened eyes, and anxiously snatched up at the first hint of a cry, you're more than likely to be an anxious adult yourself by now (which may well make you a candidate for smoking). On the other hand, if you were handled with confidence, looked at sympathetically, fed quickly when you showed signs of hunger, but not too quickly; and everything else in your little world was calm and comfortable, the chances are – that you won't be reading this!

To sum up: we inevitably come into the world complete with certain attributes, such as basic intelligence, gender, inherited characteristics, etc., but more influential than any of these in deciding our future responses and behaviour, is the style of treatment we received whilst small babies. That treatment taught us how to manage issues and feelings like those mentioned above, and that style of management in turn became a fixed part of our adult personalities. If we have not learnt how to manage such things well, we may end up particularly vulnerable to life's stresses and strains.

Stress responses and addictive behaviour

Of course that's not the beginning and end of it – if only life was that simple! There is still the question of what amounts to a stress or a strain. But that's how we develop our basic responses to, and style of coping with, the challenges of life And though styles of coping with life are hugely important for all sorts of reasons, they're absolutely critical to whether or not we choose to smoke. After all, who is more likely to end up 'needing' a mind-altering chemical: a person whose mind can cope with delay, or a person whose mind can't bear frustration?

But this is only a description of the first part of the 'something' (see page 27) that led to smoking; this is to do with the sense of self we developed as a response to our birds. There are still those 'bird droppings' to look at: the messages that gave us a set of beliefs about life and our part in it. It's when they're put together that these two set up our expectations about how life should be, and about how much 'difficult stuff' we should be able to tolerate before we feel the need, by some means of other (probably using some addictive substance or behaviour), to make the disturbing feelings go away.

Later on in the chapter we'll come back to those 'bird droppings', and to their part in influencing smoking behaviour, but first let's just think about the advantages of the idea that childhood influences lead to addictive thinking. If you can't cope with disturbing feelings when you have them (and hopefully you're not allowing yourself a negative, knee-jerk, reaction to that suggestion), don't worry, you're hardly alone: you're one of a vast group of us out there, all doing a whole lot of seriously unhealthy, unbalanced things with our lives.

Amongst all the other confusion of evidence, 'the experts' have recently come up with some research that says that people who smoke would not have had the same life expectancy or health prospects as people who've never smoked, even if they (the smokers) had never smoked. Can you manage to get your head around that? Like a lot of research around smoking it's a bit confused (not to say confusing), but it suggests that smokers belong, for some, as yet unspecified, reason, to a group of people who are fundamentally less healthy, *even before they start to smoke.*

You can accept that as it stands, and assume that if you smoke you were 'made' to do it, perhaps by something like defective genes, which also happen to make you poorer, shorter, and generally sicker in a number of ways than people who don't smoke. So there's not much you can do about it. So you might as well smoke.

Or, you can come the extra mile with me and work out that a person who's been brought up to respond poorly to life's stresses will think in unhelpful ways, including believing they need to run away from stress. That belief will lead them to search out a variety of escape routes – the sort that alter your brain chemistry, like drink, drugs, coffee, artificial foods and, of course, fags. None of which is exactly selected for its health-giving properties and all of which are addictive. The net result of all that is that addictive people in general will end up poorer, shorter, fatter, sicker, etc. And there's a good chance that they will bring up their own children in such a way that they, too, will be unable to respond well to life's stresses, so they will think in unhelpful ways too, and so on and so on.

However, the great joy in that explanation of the problem is that *it gives you control.* That's because it says if you can challenge the past and change your thinking, you can change the behaviour. Which is great news!

The bottom line, then, is that people who choose to smoke, belong to a particular category of people, not all of whom necessarily smoke, but all of whom show some form of needy or addictive behaviour as a result of early years' experience.

What links these addictive people together is that our basic response mechanisms to stimulation and stress will all be poorly adapted ones, developed at an early age. When stress and excitement hormones flood our bodies, the feelings we experience will vary from slightly to intensely uncomfortable (even when the feelings should apparently be positive ones – check the way you really feel when you're next in an exciting situation). And, because we never learnt how to manage feelings that were less than 100 per cent comfortable (and how many are?), there's no possibility of dealing with those feelings in a psychologically healthy and calm way. So what we generate in response to agitating hormones are equally agitated emotional or physical behaviours. These are ways of surviving that we learnt long, long ago; they are still quite childlike, and can look very much so from the outside. Just think of the comparison between an upset child sucking its thumb and the stressed-out adult sucking on a ciggie in a traffic jam.

That means that those of us who fit the description are likely to respond to exciting and stimulating events – such as meeting groups of new people – with excited behaviours. We are more likely to talk too much, show off, back off, or be physically twitchy or awkward, perhaps needing to hold something in our hands. We'll call those 'Type 1' responses. This is in direct contrast to the 'Type 2' response, which would be to focus on the situation and calmly discover what we can about the new people, allowing ourselves to adjust behaviour to the demands of the occasion and the personalities involved.

Equally, when faced with stressful events – such as hearing a noise in the dark – people with poor (Type 1) responses to stimulation and stress are more likely to freeze, attack the source, run away from it, gabble, cram their faces with comforting foodstuffs, have a drink, or light a fag. Type 2 responses would be to immediately assume it has some mechanical cause, work out what that might be, and decide what to do about it.

Frustratingly, if, in either kind of situation, be it exciting or frightening, people with poor responses carry out any or all, of the Type 1 things, they're going to end up activating even more of the chemicals that made them feel over-excited or desperate in the first place. So the cycle is repeated, and then you have – *addiction!*

Layers of addiction

If your instantaneous response to stimulation or stress is limited to over-acting, attacking, running or freezing, at least you aren't topping yourself up with *additional* mind-altering chemicals, and so with additional layers of addiction. If you limit yourself to those responses, you are 'simply' addicted to your own behaviour, and addiction to a behaviour can be managed in ways that aren't necessarily destructive (more on that later).

But when addictive behaviour comes with the extra 'demand' that you feed yourself with substances that are, in themselves, chemically addictive, then you have a double whammy. And herein lies the cause of what is more commonly known as addiction, that is, the seemingly unstoppable compulsion to drown your body in toxic substances, ranging from sugar and fat all the way down through fags and booze to the hardest of the hard drugs.

That unstoppable compulsion may begin with outside everyday situations, like someone offering you a cigarette, a gooey chocolate, or a joint. Some people can stop there, having just one or two. But some of us can't, and this is down to an immediate physical cause that is made up of two parts:

- A brain that has become dependent from an early age on being rewarded with instant primitive 'treats', rather than with more sophisticated longer-term satisfactions.

- A physical dependency which, once started, can only be bypassed with pain or discomfort (which an addictive person can't tolerate).

In case you think that cigarettes can't possibly be in the same league as some of the other addictions, you should know that your particular choice of toxic substance kills more people than heroin and is at least as addictive. It might also be worth knowing that recovering drug addicts and alcoholics are twice as likely to relapse if they've still kept up a smoking addiction.

What links panic reactions with booze, fags and drugs is a *mindset* that says you are only able to 'cope' with stimulation and stresses (anything from meeting new people in a social environment, to frustration at work, to divorce – with all the possibilities in between and on all the sides) by behaving in ways that will bring you shots of relief-inducing chemicals. Some of which will be internally generated, some taken in by mouth, nose or needle.

Put very, very simply, it looks like this:

- You can't/won't tolerate your own raw feelings.
- You demand something that will deflect/deaden the impact of those feelings.
- Or you run away from them.

We are about to look at the messages that tell us our feelings are so unmanageable that we need chemical help with them (and at what can be done to change all that). But first, it may comfort you to know that you're in good company.

Winston Churchill was another 'can't coper', who lived life at the extremes of feeling, and nearly drove his friends and family mad with his fluctuating moods and behaviour. His behaviour was addictive in all sorts of ways – he got over-excited, he talked too much, he ate too much and he charged madly into any and every activity. He also suffered deep depressions (which he called his 'Black Dog'), which repeatedly led him to think of suicide. To top it all off, his addictive behaviour demanded the next layer – chemical addiction – and he smoked and drank, virtually non-stop. He may, somehow, have managed to stay in charge of the country, but he never quite managed to stay in charge of himself and his own moods. He never dealt with the chemical rushes of stimulation and stress without falling back on addictive behaviours and substances. If it hadn't been for the overwhelming demands of politics and war, who knows how he might have ended up? What we do know, though, is that he had a childhood lacking in empathy and warmth.

And then there are all those lesser celebrities, the artists, actors and models whose troubled lives seem to fill newspapers, magazines and TV reality shows, and who seem to fluctuate between wanting attention and wanting 'to be alone'. The ones whose lives are punctuated by highs, lows and time spent in clinics. When they're photographed 'in the raw', isn't it funny how often they seem to have fags in hand? Going back to the idea of smokers' fantasies that I mentioned in the first chapter, are those really the fags of creativity or fun? Or are they the fags of the neediness, which wafts in clouds around attention-seekers, and which drives them to all kinds of Type 1 behaviour, and especially to addiction to chemical substances?

The role of nicotine in addiction

Sadly, the truth is that the nicotine in cigarettes really does feel like a helper if you're needy. Nicotine can help to focus thoughts – if they're pretty unfocused to start with. It can help calm people down – if they're over-excited to start with. It can make us feel better – if we feel bad to start with. But nicotine is an evil little substance in more ways than one. Because the other effect that nicotine has is *to stimulate*.

You (or Churchill, or Famous Ms X) get all stressed or excited, feel you need calming, so you smoke a cigarette, feel calmer, and able to think more clearly. But then, blow me if you don't feel all needy again, and the thing you're in need of is ... another cigarette – to calm you down again! Any relief you got was only temporary. Like sympathetic kidnappers who make us feel grateful for the five minutes' occasional exercise they give us in exchange for our freedom, cigarettes make us value five minutes' clearer thinking more than the long-term use of a body and brain with unclogged lungs and arteries. Or they would, if it weren't for the fact that, in themselves, cigarettes are nothing at all. Until we choose to smoke them. And how clear can anyone's thinking be when they make that choice? It's a no-brainer!

A drug to get off drugs

It's ironic that an anti-depressant, Zyban, is often used to help people quit smoking. If you think about it, anyone who smokes is already hooked on using chemicals to change their moods, so can another drug to unhook ourselves, albeit a benevolent one, be the best way to tackle our problem?

It's better by far to deal with the addictive neediness itself and the thinking that underlies it: to 're-programme' ourselves so that we learn to cope with life all by ourselves.

Programming and re-programming

So, let's go back to finding out why you ended up programmed to over-respond to aspects of life in the particular way you do at the moment. And after that we'll concentrate on why you choose to use cigarettes as one of your addictive responses.

When we come into the world, we have certain attributes already in place, such as basic intelligence, gender and inherited characteristics, and it seems that sometimes these will include a greater than normal susceptibility to developing addictive behaviours. For example, people with autistic tendencies, or naturally high levels of certain hormones (such as testosterone), or lower than average IQs, may be more at risk of dependency generally. This doesn't mean that they will inevitably become ˉaddicts; but since they may be less skilled than others at analysing their own behaviour or at coping with stress, they will be particularly vulnerable to addiction. However, allowing for such exceptions, for the great majority of us the most significant factor affecting the chances of our becoming addicted remains our experiences in childhood.

The best experiences in childhood (and we are talking perfection here) include such consistently sympathetic and empathetic care that a baby can develop the capacity to manage its feelings and cope (in simple ways) with excitement, distress and frustration. Confident handling and good mental and physical stimulation are an important part of the equation, too. But there is even more: a baby also needs to discover, at the very simplest of levels, how to be satisfied with being its own person. If a baby can occasionally find amusement in watching shadows move, rather than needing always to be entertained, it will learn how to be at peace with itself. So, in addition to stimulation babies also need space and time to relax. Space and time when they're not fussed and over-managed, and can develop early responsibility for their feelings.

Parents don't always come with PhDs in childcare, so sometimes they get bits of this complex job wrong. And then children's ways of coping end up a bit wrong, too. We've seen how they might end up feeling insecure and needy for attention, angry a lot of the time, or unable to tolerate frustration. But you've probably already realised that you know lots of non-smokers who have inadequate coping skills. Inadequate coping skills in themselves don't necessarily result in any very specific behaviours. They might make someone grumpy, jumpy and anxious, but they won't *inevitably* lead to addiction to substances. There's another part of the 'something' (which comes between birth and the first cigarette) to fill in before we can get the full picture of how addiction comes about.

Bird droppings as messages

The second part of the 'something' comes in the form of the little bombs that those birds I mentioned earlier dropped down on us. The 'droppings' that landed, splat, on those little pink babies, who were already busy developing specific coping responses, were the first messages we heard about ourselves and life.

These messages will have come in the form of comments like:
'Always such a good little girl, no bother at all.'
'Nobody wants to play with somebody who won't share their toys.'
'Why does everything always go wrong?'
'Oh, go on, have a little ciggie. It'll help you relax.'

And these seemingly insignificant messages, when they are repeated and confirmed often enough, actually do teach us what we should think about ourselves and expect from ourselves or from life in general.

So, to add to the coping responses that have left us less than great at coping with our feelings in certain situations, we are now looking to find the early messages that have led to us being more likely to deal with the resulting neediness (or emptiness or excitability) created by life's little stresses and strains by giving in to it (as in sucking a ciggie to achieve its nicotine 'calm'), rather than by holding it in check.

Messages in action

It's all very well talking hypothetically, but let's put arms and legs on the ways that a poorly developed coping mechanism might get topped up by certain types of bird droppings and lead to a child developing expectations of itself and life that could lead to addiction. Here are some imaginary, but typical, scenarios:

Example 1

A young mum takes her toddler daughter, Ellie, into the supermarket and there in front of Ellie as she goes in is a packet of lovely pink and white marshmallows. She loves marshmallows and doesn't like having to wait for anything, so she immediately demands them. At first she's given the answer, 'No', so Ellie bursts into hysterical tears (already not good at dealing with frustration). Mum then quickly gives in, and not only puts the sweets in the trolley, but actually lets Ellie eat some from the packet as she's going around the supermarket.

On top of that, within Ellie's earshot, Mum says to the girl at the check-out, 'Little so and so, she never could wait for anything.' And there you have it! Every minute of that seemingly innocent shopping trip taught Ellie to think of herself as someone who couldn't, and shouldn't, have to wait to gratify her appetite. She learnt to think of herself in terms of 'I must have what I want, when I want, no matter if it's not good for me, otherwise it's okay if I throw some kind of hissy fit'.

And later, when Ellie grows up, she will probably still want to have what she wants when she wants it, even if it's likely to kill her, and never mind the effect it's going to have on the people all around her.

Example 2

Little Darren, who has never learnt to manage frustration, is playing with another tot, who doesn't hand over a toy quickly enough for Darren's liking. So he whacks him. Darren's Mum (or Dad, or Auntie, let's not always blame Mum) turns straight to the other kid's Mum and says, 'Your Johnnie must have hit my little Darren first – he's not one to do anything like that.'

The message Little Darren learns about himself and life from this episode is that he's the kind of person who's allowed to get away with things. He has allowances made for him, he doesn't have to take responsibility and can see himself (unreasonably) as a victim, even of his own frustration, rather than as a bully.

Darren will probably grow up blaming everything and everyone but himself for his problems, and more to the point, running away from any prospect of accepting blame, possibly using chemical substances as an escape route.

Example 3

Mr and Mrs Nice and their three oldest children feel they should always 'protect' the family 'baby' from anything nasty. So when the family cat dies, all the older members of the family pretend that it has simply 'gone away'. As the baby grows up, the family, without meaning any harm, not only keep her permanently immature and dependent but also drop the message that for some chosen people, such as her, reality is far too overwhelming to be dealt with. When crises happen, the best thing to do is to deny them all round.

In later life that youngest child may find it easier to hide from unpleasant reality behind chemical fingers.

Example 4

Charlie is anxious for her Dad's attention and approval. One fine summer's day Charlie asks Dad if they can play footie together in the park, but Dad says, 'Are you kidding? Forget it, there's a big match on the box. But if you're quiet you can sit in.' So the child obediently forgets it, and joins Dad and his beer in the darkened lounge. There they both lie flat out on the settee watching telly through the long, hot, afternoon. What does a kid like Charlie learn from that? That to be acceptable she must live life on the sidelines and watch it go by?

When Charlie grows up, rather than enjoying and respecting her body, she is more likely to treat it like a binbag for chemical rubbish.

Picking up your own messages

With so many different messages out there and so many ways of picking them up, it's highly unlikely yours will fit any of these patterns exactly. The most important thing to focus on is what you ended up believing about yourself and about how you should deal with life. And somewhere or other, in amongst the messages that addictive people pick up, there will have been very particular ones, which led to attitudes that are:

- Judgmental, critical, perfectionist.

- Self-indulgent, body-abusing.

- People-pleasing, easily led, self-critical, self-pitying, depressed.

- Resentful, awkward, rebellious, grandiose.

- Risk-taking, sensation-seeking or any of the other attitudes that usually go with smoking behaviour.

Your attitudes to yourself and life

The check-list below will help you define those attitudes. When you read each statement, consider whether it applies to or describes your attitudes, your ways of dealing with life. If you recognise it as something that you think or say, tick the box. Try to see yourself as if from the outside, and be really ruthless about yourself when you choose the appropriate answers. It's important to be as objective and honest as possible.

I need what I need and I always need it immediately.	☐
I can't bear pain/frustration/excitement (or any other 'overdose' of sensation) and I shouldn't have to.	☐
I need constant excitement and stimulation. I must never feel bored, or be left with nothing to do but twiddle my thumbs and reflect on life.	☐
I need soothing, I should always feel calm. It's not good for me to feel agitated.	☐

Nobody tells me what to do. * ☐

I can't be alone. ☐

I don't like myself. ☐

I should have what I want because I'm worth it. ☐

I should have what I want because I'll feel unloved without it. ☐

I should have what I want because I'll feel a failure without it. ☐

* That attitude is a sentence to a lifetime of ignorance and stupidity if you think about it, yet it's one that is common to smokers.

Now, finish the unfinished comments below in your own words (the ideas in brackets are merely suggestions). Think long and hard about the truth in each case. And make sure you write down all your answers, either here, or on a separate sheet of paper.

Note: If when you're thinking about any of the examples you can hear a tiny voice deep inside you muttering, 'Otherwise it's just not fair or right!', then you'll know that's the give-away, telling you that this particular attitude began in early childhood. Think of the examples of Ellie and Charlie and tell the story of a particular episode from your own life that would perfectly explain how it might have come about.

When I'm angry I should … (let rip, bottle my feelings up)

When I'm anxious I should … (feel ill, let everyone know)

When I'm relaxing I should … (feed my appetites, switch off from people)

I have a right to feel … (guilt free, comfortable, happy)

When I'm working/being creative I need to feel ... (on edge, twitchy, manic)

```
┌─────────────────────────────────────────────────────────┐
│                                                         │
│                                                         │
└─────────────────────────────────────────────────────────┘
```

In order to feel really alive I need ... (to live life on the edge, to feel rebellious)

```
┌─────────────────────────────────────────────────────────┐
│                                                         │
│                                                         │
└─────────────────────────────────────────────────────────┘
```

In order to feel really appreciated I need ... (to have attention, to be gratified)

```
┌─────────────────────────────────────────────────────────┐
│                                                         │
│                                                         │
└─────────────────────────────────────────────────────────┘
```

When quite juvenile attitudes such as these get bolted on to a basic coping mechanism that is also immature, we're going to find ourselves perfectly programmed to over-respond to some aspects of life. The situation will contain the perfect cocktail of characteristics to encourage us to feel that we're in need of some sort of physical reward, compensation or stimulant to keep us going while facing life's stresses and strains.

But having got this far through the book you – and your attitudes – should be maturing fast! And you should be taking personal responsibility for your smoking as you recognise that all the things which we think of as 'making' us smoke are really only happening *in our own heads*. They're not outside forces at all: they are simply long-established feelings that have been made irresistible by fixed sets of attitudes telling us what we should think about those feelings.

And there lie the root causes of your smoking behaviour.

So now we've got to the origins of the needy feeling and of the permission we give ourselves to indulge it that are the foundations of addictive behaviour. But we're not yet quite at the point of identifying the day-to-day triggers that result in your feeling the need for chemical support. Nor have we discovered the reasons why it's a pack of cigarettes that you reach for. That's all to come.

In the next chapter we're going to work out what are the circumstances that can still inappropriately stimulate or aggravate that old needy feeling in your modern world. Through this, you will learn to recognise those circumstances in the future when they crop up, and to be on your guard against further self-harm.

Then we can start the re-programming of the way you react to stresses of one sort or another, and challenge the old trigger moments that used to have you reaching for that cardboard carton full of tubes of toxicity.

All the way to the end, keep on reminding yourself:

- Smoking is just a series of actions that you carry out.

- No series of actions that you voluntarily perform is *ever* really out of your control.

- And we shouldn't forget that there is *no* cigarette, even the odd one that we have, 'just to be sociable with my mates on a Friday night,' that could ever be said to be harmless. How can any of us know which cigarette is the one that's going to tip the balance of our cells' health towards cancer?

Mix and Match

Or, Identifying the trigger moment

We are now going to start looking for the connection between your personality and the root causes of your smoking behaviour, using the answers you gave to the mini-questionnaires starting on page 15 (the ones which described that behaviour in detail). Once this is done, you'll be in a good position to identify your own particular trigger moments, which lead to smoking.

When we see how our early coping skills and consequent ways of reacting to life are mirrored in our current smoking behaviour, we start to understand what goes into each individual decision we take to smoke a cigarette. We need to be able to recognise those specific triggers that are likely to set off that smoking behaviour at any given time before we can break the chain reaction. Recognising what the triggers consist of is the equivalent of knowing the settings of a time bomb. This is vital: if we don't know what the settings are, we can't prevent the bomb going off, however much we might want to, or however hard we might try.

Back to the questionnaires

First we are going to try to identify any patterns of behaviour that you show. The answers you gave to the three separate sets of questions will give you three informal sets of information about your smoking behaviour. These consist of:

- The various patterns and ceremonials of your behaviour when buying and smoking cigarettes
- The rewards you feel you get from the behaviour
- Your earliest experience of the behaviour.

Pull out the papers you wrote your answers down on. (And if you haven't got them, that in itself should tell you something...) Look at your answers again but this time analyse them piece by piece, in minute detail. Think like a forensic pathologist and do your own post mortem on the body of evidence.

Patterns

Take a look at the first set of answers to see what you can find out about yourself. Are you careful or impulsive, dirty or tidy, driven or lazy, greedy or sparing? What kind of person are you describing in those answers, and what does what you've written about your ceremonials tell you about your priorities and standards? If, for example, you've said you have no idea how much you spend on indulgences like smoking, that could suggest you prioritise personal appetite over family responsibility. If that were true, what would knowing that tell you about your specific neediness and about when it's likely to overwhelm you?

And although this is jumping the gun rather, here's something to consider as you go along: is there anything in that information you've given in the questionnaire to suggest how you might start breaking any of your patterns of behaviour? It doesn't have to be anything complicated – so could you swap from a lighter to matches, for instance, or from holding cigarettes in the right hand to the left?

Rewards

The answers to the first set of questions starting on page 15 dealt with reasonably straightforward material, but those you gave in your responses on pages 20–21 will give you subtler information, so you'll need to analyse them even more closely. For example, if you said that one of the emotional rewards you got from smoking was 'feeling defiant', the most obvious conclusion from that is that you're a bit of a rebel. Hardly insightful and you probably know it already. If you dig deeper for clues though, another, more useful picture emerges, this time of someone who's felt so dominated by a person or situation in their past that they're no longer completely free to be themselves. They've become more focused on reacting *against* their world than on developing a mature and independent relationship with it.

This second way of seeing yourself might be less sexy, but it could be more constructive. You're much more likely to want to dispose of unhelpful and regressive feelings if you think they make you look sad rather than feisty. And if you can dispose of them, the smoking behaviour they've led to will follow suit.

Early experiences

Your answers to the third set of questions (on pages 22–24), which ask you about the time you first started smoking, will identify the external influences that led up to that first cigarette and the state of mind you were in when you had it. But they will also throw up another question: 'Every time you light up in the here and now, do you either want or need to turn the clock back and revisit your own past?'

The information about early smoking behaviour is really significant. Where we were, who we were with, who knew about the cigarettes, whether they disapproved of them, how we felt about ourselves, whether we were ashamed, scared etc. is all important and relevant. So don't rush past this section. Take Sidney as a case study.

Sidney smoked his first cigarette to prove to his tough friends that he wasn't a wimp, and to prove to himself that he was one of the gang. But he smoked it crouching in his friend's father's potting shed, terrified he was going to be caught any minute. Sidney is now a 20-a-day smoker, and every one of those cigarettes is nailing that original state of mind more firmly in place, because every time Sidney has one he remembers the sense of shame, fear and worthlessness as an ongoing feeling deep inside. Each cigarette prevents him freeing himself from childhood chains.

A picture of you

Overall, some picture or pattern of behaviour will emerge from these answers. Imagine that you have to write a screenplay and want to depict a character through their behaviour. You know that the occasions they choose to light up and the way they smoke their cigarettes is going to say more to the audience about their state of mind and intentions than any number of words. From the evidence that you've given about your own habits, there would be enough information for the director and cameraman to show you as a very detailed character, with very specific behaviour. Can you see all that for yourself, yet?

We already know that, whatever information you might have given about yourself, the cameraman won't be zooming in on a person in a state of complete grace. However calm smokers may believe themselves to be whilst they're puffing away, the reality is that their bodies are under constant chemical assault, and so, during waking hours, they can never be totally relaxed. They will usually be working themselves up to the next cigarette, therefore they are more or less permanently in a state of expectancy, even if they have learnt to call some part of this state relaxation. True relaxation can (and will) only come once the nicotine addiction and the behavioural addiction are in the past.

The good news is that, as you read on, with each page you read you will be working your way towards that true state of healthful calm. Each reflection on your old thoughts and behaviour is counting out the old needs and counting in the new mindset. You're in the act of building your future as you read.

Getting in touch with your senses

So now we've established your pattern of behaviour. In the last chapter you'd already worked out where your neediness comes from and you've also looked at the attitudes (the result of the bird droppings) which allow you to give in to neediness, rather than defy it. Can you see now how the patterns of our actual, real-time, everyday behaviour reflect both our neediness and our attitudes? That, for example, if we've had a childhood which left us forever striving for perfection but feeling inadequate in the lovability stakes, as adults we might well need to define ourselves by the smooth running and success of our personal relationships. And if we then have a blazing row with a lover, we are likely to reflect all our past neediness and attitudes in the way we buy ten fags and then smoke them all, one after another, greedily, tidily but secretly, in a back lane. But we may not feel a need to smoke again until the next time we have a row that stirs up all those old ghosts.

Of course it's that word, 'feel', that's the key word. Feel the need. Near the start of this book I said that it's not the feelings themselves that count, so much as the thoughts that we have about the feelings. That remains the case throughout life and, as we've seen over and over again, the thoughts we have come about as a result of our attitudes, etc. However, what we're going to need to focus on now is the 'structure' of the feeling itself. It's all very well talking about feelings, but what do we mean by 'feelings'? What does a feeling *feel* like?

I could write about them being combinations of sensations and thoughts, but we're not about to go into philosophical labyrinths here! It's enough for the purposes of this book to describe them as bodily sensations that we learn to associate with certain emotional states. And – here's the clever bit – we can use them as signposts for the direction our behaviour is *about to* go in.

When it comes to the question of smoking, feelings work this way: we experience a set of physical sensations (courtesy of all those chemicals, hormones, etc.) as a response to certain circumstances, then we think, 'Oh, no. Can't cope with that, I need to feel calmer,' so we light a fag, feel calmer ... and then go round the loop again, as we've seen before. But if we can learn to recognise what the physical sensations are that *lead to* that loop, we can also recognise the circumstances that give rise to the sensations in the first place. It's chicken and egg, but if we can avoid or neutralise either the feelings or the circumstances, we won't follow through with the behaviour.

What do the feelings feel like?

You need now to 'go back into' the feelings you have *before* you smoke. To do this effectively, don't smoke the next few cigarettes that you would usually expect to have. Let your need for a cigarette build up, so that you can then really get to grips with the physical sensations you're experiencing. We're often really bad at knowing our own bodies, so try to do a complete body check on yourself, work out what is going on in minute physical detail, to the point where you end up knowing the feeling so intimately you could recognise its breathing in the dark!

Speaking of which, when you feel the need for a cigarette, how is your breathing? Try running that body check:

- Is your breathing shallow, exaggerated, quick?

- Where is physical tension located? Is it in your shoulders, back, tummy ... where?

- How does your face feel? Your brow? Your jaw?

- What does your head feel like on the inside?

- What are your hands and feet doing?

- What are you experiencing in the middle area of your body, inside in your abdomen?

- What other sensations are you experiencing?

- Is there a particular point at which that set of bodily sensations, that feeling, really does start to seem overwhelming? And with hindsight, would that be the very point when your conscious brain starts to disengage and your hand just finds itself full of cigarette?

If that is the case then you have found your 'trigger feeling' – and that leads straight to the trigger moment, which is simply the moment when all the right circumstances come together to trigger that feeling, the one that is the forerunner to the cigarette.

At last we're getting there! Once we've caught the trigger moment, we mustn't let it go. We need to remind ourselves what it feels like from time to time, so that we'll recognise it when it steals up on us. And that will always be the time when we're most vulnerable to relapse, so it's important for each of us to work out what actually makes up our own particular trigger moments.

Ingredients of the trigger moment

The ingredients of a trigger moment are a complete soup. There isn't a set recipe, nor do all the ingredients always have to be in place for the mix to work. On one day it might take only one of the ingredients to set us off smoking; but on another day when we are stronger, less vulnerable, it might need every one of them to be in place before that ancient sense of neediness that creates that trigger feeling is sparked off. For any one of us there will be a variety of things involved but, by and large, the type of ingredient in our trigger moment will come from certain basic categories. These include:

- Situation

- Location

- People

- Emotional circumstances

- Sensory details, like smell, sound, etc.

And once these ingredients have been hard-wired inside us, they will always have the power to set off that trigger feeling which is associated with our need for addictive behaviour and substances. (There will be more about why we've chosen cigarettes as our particular, if not only, addictive substance later.)

No hierarchies apply here. A seemingly insignificant circumstance may have as great an effect on one person as an obviously calamitous set of circumstances on someone else. It might take the death of a parent to get one person reaching for a pack of cigarettes, whilst it is enough for another to be held up in a traffic jam. We're not talking weakness or judgement here, merely individual cause and effect.

That probably makes it sound as though most smokers only smoke under extreme pressure, which, as we all know, is obviously not so. Most smokers get into a habit of smoking, often when they don't in fact feel like it. When you're working out the ingredients of your trigger moments, don't worry too much about all those odd unconsidered cigarettes (though aren't they all!), concentrate on the ones you really felt you *needed;* the use of that word 'need' is all-important. All the others will only be pale reflections of those anyway. Then consider how the individual ingredients from that short list might combine in your case.

Situation
This may be one of the most powerful of the ingredients. Perhaps we're having to deal with an elusive supplier of goods, or organise an important event, go to a social function, take over the running of a workforce, look after someone sick, accept criticism, get out of a relationship, walk home in the dark, go to court, cope with a death, sit with a drink, fly on a plane, deal with a teenager. These are all typical situations in which smokers 'feel the need' for a cigarette. Yours may be like none of these. But whatever they are, you need to know which particular situations leave you 'feeling in need' of a cigarette.

Location
This needn't be as precise as, say, Brighton seafront, but it may be as particular as, 'in my office', or, 'only ever on the loo'. For most of us it's probably going to be more like, 'Well, I'd say anywhere, but if I'm ruthless, it's actually anywhere that isn't in a vehicle, in someone's house, or out and about in the centre of town.' Which is quite precise if you think about it. So, how precise can you be about the location of your trigger moments?

People
This might mean that you smoke in the company of your mates, or only ever in the relative anonymity of a crowded city centre pub. On the other hand, it might mean you choose to smoke while not actually in the company of someone, but whilst seeing them in your mind. For example, if we smoke after a row with a partner or a friend, then that person is probably featuring in a little film that we're running in our mind's eye. What matters is whether a person, or sets of people, feature regularly in your smoking behaviour. Do you have trigger moments when very particular people feature in your life, either in person, or when you're thinking of them?

Emotional circumstances

This is arguably the most powerful ingredient of all, and in a way everything in this book relates to this. After all, as I have said repeatedly, if we have always felt okay about ourselves, and continue to do so, how can we have any reason to want to poison ourselves just so that we can manage our feelings? However, we can think of emotional circumstances in a more limited way as part of this list of ingredients – as the emotional background or stage set, in front of which all the other circumstances might be gathering. So, if boyfriend Jason is up there in the people role, and the location is the bench in the park where you always meet, and the situation is that you had an argument earlier on the phone and are now going to try to patch things up, what are the emotional circumstances of this occasion going to be? And you can always add or subtract intensity if there have been other events, such as tension at work, or a little win on the lottery, that are likely to affect your emotions. The big question is, what are our presiding emotional states when we feel most *in need of a cigarette?* Are they evidently upset ones, or perhaps ones that are slightly hyper?

Sensory details

These may seem relatively unimportant, unless you remember Noel Coward's words about never underestimating the power of cheap music. In fact, all kinds of sounds, like music, and all kinds of smells, like perfume or school dinners, can whizz us back to past times faster than you can say 'quicksticks'. And if it weren't for the fact that hardened smokers lose their powers of smell to a great extent, the impact would probably be bigger still. Are particular smells, noises, or sights likely to trigger off your desire for a ciggie? And what about a combination of all three, say the hoppy scent, the whishing sound and the sight of the foaming head of a pint of beer being pulled?

If thinking about all these details has actually whetted your desire to light up or – even worse – actually sent you off in search of a pack of 20, there is something positive that you can take from that: which is the more precise understanding you now have of just what it is that sets you going. But never lose sight of the fact that what sets you going is not actually to do with the outside factors themselves (after all, they probably repulse somebody else) but to do with the way you *feel* about them. And the way you feel about things is all down to the coping strategies and attitudes you have learned. Remember?

Keeping tempting thoughts out of mind is not the only, or necessarily the best, way of dealing with them. In due course we're going to look at ways of immersing ourselves in them and learning how to deal differently with them, so that they lose the power to affect us. In the meantime, tempting thoughts are sources of information about our vulnerabilities.

Learning from the patterns

When we look at the patterns of our smoking behaviour, all the way through, from its beginning right up to now, we can learn various things from those patterns.

- That our early learned attitudes and ways of coping are reflected both in our need to smoke and in the particular ways we smoke

- That the times we most need to smoke are when our old ways of feeling from the past are stimulated in the present; these are our 'trigger feelings'

- That the circumstances when these crop up can be broken down into times, places, situations, etc., which, when they come together, produce our trigger moments for addictive needs, which in turn lead to smoking

- That the circumstances that produce these very powerful feelings need to be understood and recognised because these will be the ones most likely to cause a relapse after quitting

- That recognising the chain of cause and effect is central to quitting smoking.

We haven't yet spent very much time looking at how this all fits into the actual strategies you can use to make the quitting process easier and more positive, but that is, of course, central to your reason for reading this, or any other, book about giving up smoking. You want to make quitting as painless to yourself as possible. I made a couple of suggestions earlier, which start to show how information you discover about your smoking behaviour itself, and about your underlying reasons for it, can be converted into strategies to help you with the quitting process. Each new piece of information about the background to your smoking can be worked with positively to give you a new 'tool' for quitting.

There will be whole chapters devoted to this later, but it can only be helpful to start thinking along those lines as you go. So from here on, think about what any neediness you might be feeling could really indicate. That cigarette you think you need is nothing in itself, it is a symbol, something that takes the place of something else. Start to look at alternatives to fulfil the 'need'. If you're feeling unloved, wouldn't a hug be better than a cigarette? Okay, okay, so you're sitting in a traffic jam. Find your own suggestions.

Your story so far

In the next chapter we're going to move on to the specific reasons you have for choosing cigarettes as your particular addictive behaviour and chemical, but before we do, this is a good time to do a quick inventory of what you have discovered about yourself so far. It will help to keep the process that lies behind addiction in mind, so that we don't forget that smoking is not an inevitability, but an outcome of very particular factors that have come together in our lives. And it will also help to remind us that, whatever those past factors might have been, we should by now be free to make choices more in line with what we want for ourselves today.

So, let's go through that inventory.

You might find it easier, or quicker, to put this into a mental slide show or video, or you may prefer just to work with a series of data.

Consider

- What unreal or fantasy images you may have held of yourself or smoking before you started reading this book

- The detailed picture of the various elements of your smoking behaviour, looked at from the outside in

- The ways you might assess the smoking behaviour if you were looking at it as an outsider.

Take into account

- Your first experiences in life as a child and the coping skills you developed in response to them

- The early childhood messages you learned about yourself and life and the attitudes you developed from these

- The emotional neediness you felt as a child, and may show in certain pre-addictive behaviours

- The circumstances and experience of that first cigarette, or early smoking behaviour

- What or whom that cigarette was to satisfy

- The elements of the 'trigger feeling' that are associated with the need for subsequent cigarettes

- The circumstances that give rise to it and which, with it, provide the trigger moment which, so far, has been irresistible.

Good. With that picture of yourself in mind we can now move on, from the causes of addictive thinking and behaviour, to the specific addiction itself.

Finally, we are coming to the very obvious question, 'Why do you smoke cigarettes?'

It's a Fag

Or, Why cigarettes are your substance of choice

Many a person writing a book about quitting smoking would be starting here, because this section of the book is going to take a look at the reasons smokers smoke cigarettes. For some people, this is the most significant factor in giving up smoking – working out what you get from a ciggie and then saying how you can learn to live without it. As though what you get from a cigarette has an independent and magnetic quality all of its own.

What that approach completely fails to take into account is the fact that cigarettes provide what they provide regardless of whether or not you choose to smoke them. They sit there on the shelf in the newsagents, in huge containerloads by the ferry terminal, in silver cigarette cases, and in the overpriced pub vending machine, completely unconcerned, oblivious to your very existence even. How can cigarettes provide any incentives to you to smoke them? They are what they are; some people use them, some people don't, so it can hardly be claimed that their charms are irresistible. Whatever a cigarette has to offer, that in itself is no explanation of why a person would choose to be associated with it. A prostitute in PVC will only appeal to people who have a taste for both prostitutes and PVC.

So, at the risk of becoming a bore, I will stress yet again that the underlying reason for anyone to smoke cigarettes is to be found in the head of the smoker and not in the cigarettes themselves. Which is the underlying reason that we have concentrated on looking inside our own heads first, rather than at what cigarettes, in themselves, 'have to offer'. But we've now got to the point at which it has finally become relevant to ask why, given that we are needy, and wanting to use stimulants and relaxants, we should choose cigarettes as our preferred service providers.

Cigarettes or smoking?

Which of these are you giving up? Some people will say one and some the other. Which camp do you fall into? Perhaps neither? Perhaps you will say it depends, according to your mood. And yet there is a difference: cigarettes are the physical objects we use, but smoking is the action we carry out. So, if we think about it carefully, the way we choose to visualise what we're doing will tell us quite a lot about our sense of involvement in the process. It's perhaps easier to give up objects than it is to stop doing something habitual.

Either way, when we quit we get a double bonus because we've succeeded in disposing of two unwanted birds with one stone.

First, we will have put firmly into the past expensive and unlovely objects that have served only one purpose, which was to carry toxins into our systems.

And second, we will have put behind us behaviour which only led to dependency, addiction and, ultimately, damage to our health.

But that is moving ahead rather quickly. Before we get to our personal outcome of giving up cigarettes and smoking, we've still to see where they have fitted into our lives, and what they have 'provided' for us. And to do that we need first to have a little bit of context, to see where they have fitted into society generally.

An extremely brief and eccentric history of smoking and cigarettes

Tobacco was brought to Europe from the Americas (where it was thought by the indigenous people to have medicinal qualities) in the 1550s, but by 1611 the English king, James 1, was already writing that its use (in pipes) was a vile custom and came from corrupted baseness. There was never a European 'golden age' when smoking was universally accepted and approved of. But smokers haven't always known about the downsides and dangers of smoking and then chosen to ignore them either. It's more the case that, until fairly recently (in historical terms), people were scientifically and medically naive, and believed, along with the original native smokers, that smoking killed germs, and while occasionally offensive, could actually be good for their health. When cigarettes took over in popularity from other forms of smoking, manufacturers (surprise, surprise) went out of their way to encourage the health implications, whilst challenging the idea that they might be in any way offensive.

And by 1910 a brand of cigarette was being advertised in this fascinating way (eat your heart out Saatchi and Saatchi!):

> *Is it true you haven't tried it?*
> *Why! there's none can stand beside it,*
> *It's the softest and the sweetest you can get.*
> *Though our climate may be murkish*
> *You can draw delight quite Turkish,*
> *By smoking the* El Hamur *cigarette.*
> *And if your wife should clamour*
> *For a pull at your* El Hamur
> *O, Satisfy her craving, little pet!*
> *For one thing's very certain –*
> *It won't hang about the curtain,*
> *So she'll worship your* El Hamur *cigarette.*
> *Then take a match and light one,*
> *And you'll find it quite the right one,*
> *And thro' life you'll smoke no other one you bet!*
> *And when dying, you will stammer –*
> *'Oh where is my* El Hamur?
> *'My* El Hamur, *my* El Hamur *cigarette?'*

Which suggests, if we consider all the poem's implications, that these particular cigarettes were good not only for health, but also for home and marriage! Making them a domestic and marital necessity, even though the poem ends, rather poignantly, with the death of its smoker husband/hero!

What the poem also highlights, though, is the existence of a gender gap in smoking at that time. Tobacco, in the form it was originally used, in pipes or in cigars, had never been considered a suitable indulgence for respectable women. However healthful it might have been for tough men, it was also strong and smelly, and its use was connected with the all male culture found in taverns and coffee houses where commercial and political deals were done. Some women made it their business to rebel against the stereotypes that kept them weak and dependent and so they smoked as part of their rebellion, for example, the nineteenth-century French poet George Sand adopted a man's name, men's suits and cigars. But for most women it wasn't until cigarettes took over in popularity from cigars, somewhere around the turn of the nineteenth and twentieth centuries that smoking became 'dainty' enough for them.

And what becomes clear from the advert for the all-conquering 'El Hamur', is that by 1910 women were finally beginning to be recognised as potential consumers (and, of course, buyers) of cigarettes. From then it was only going to be a matter of time (the First World War, 1914 to 1918, in fact) before they were seeing themselves as being at least as entitled to smoke as men had been in the past. Smoking was quickly becoming a feminist issue.

During the First World War women took on all kinds of work and activities that had previously been thought of as 'for men only'. And when it was over they did not suddenly decide to give them all up. So working in offices, driving cars, going out alone and of course smoking came to be seen as part of the brave new world of emancipated young women, or flappers, as they were called. But it wasn't just for flappers that smoking represented part of a new, freer world, and in the 1920s smoking became accepted by nearly all of Western society, as one of the great liberties of the modern age. It was promoted by advertisers as being sophisticated, soothing, healthy and a friend in times of need, and it became the prop of choice of a thousand sultry and charismatic movie stars. There was nothing that a cigarette couldn't add to your life in the 1920s and '30s, it seemed.

During the Second World War cigarettes were even doled out with the rations of serving men and women. They were seen as supplying an essential comfort to people who were either bored out of their brains or terrified out of their wits for most of the time. And, in the films which were made during the war, cigarettes took on the twin supporting roles of doctor and therapist, as they were given to the wounded and smoked to overcome grief.

Given the near universal supply of cigarettes during the war and the positive encouragement to smoke them, it's hardly surprising that, by the end of it, smoking had become just a fact of life for millions. The lucky ones were the many thousands who had no underlying reason to have a substantial addiction to cigarettes, but had simply developed a longstanding habit coupled with the usual short-term chemical dependency. They were the ones who were able to stop smoking like a shot when the earliest convincing evidence came out which linked smoking to all sorts of ill health.

And gradually, through the 1950s to the present day, more and more research was done that linked smoking to cancer, heart disease and strokes, but you already know all about that, so I won't go over it again here.

Over the last few years a big shift has taken place in the attitude of both media and pundits and it's been in a direction away from smoking and away from believing it can be thought of as an acceptable social habit. Things have now moved so far that smoking has actually become a pariah habit, not only silently disapproved of, as it might have been in the past, but actively and loudly criticised, which certainly wasn't the case. But the movement on the ground hasn't been an equal one because it has largely taken place among the middle classes, the employed and people over 30. They are the ones who have taken on board all the new messages from the pundits and the media.

Sadly, the same can't be said of the other groups and especially of younger people. They seem to have avoided or ignored the messages and can hardly be said to believe that smoking is a pariah habit if – as is happening – they are taking it up nearly as fast as ever. Even more significant than that, probably, is the fact that, having taken it up, they are then failing to give it up in anything like the same numbers as older people. Whatever is going on?

I said earlier that smoking became a feminist issue at the start of the twentieth century. At the time, it seemed as if the right to smoke was linked to women's fight for the vote, as if it represented part of their enfranchisement. And whatever the sanity of using a cancer stick as a weapon in the war of independence, from that fight for women's emancipation onwards, cigarette smoking seems to have symbolised people's rejection of unreasonable authority.

Since it's now teenagers who appear to have assumed the role of being unreasonably put upon and disenfranchised by authority (as they see it), they've also taken enthusiastically to the use of cigarettes to symbolise their rejection.

And of course, once they've started smoking ...!

But there are two big differences between the feminists and the teenagers. The first is that feminists didn't know about all the dangers of smoking back in the early part of the twentieth century and young people nowadays have health messages drummed into them wherever they turn. So whatever is it that makes so many of these younger people ignore all the evidence and risk the danger to their health just so they can experience the joy of rebellion?

Well, it's long been a truth universally acknowledged that, courtesy of all those hormones which are sloshing around inside them, teenagers are generally bolshie and rather unco-operative. Which means they will always get a kind of perverse satisfaction from doing pretty much the opposite of whatever they are advised to do by authority figures, however sensible, well-meaning, or even in their own immediate interests that advice might be. For example, even an enticement such as, 'If you promise me you'll never smoke I'll buy you a new computer,' will rarely cut much ice with teenagers. Added to which, their pleasure in rebellion will be even greater if their behaviour can in any way be defined as 'cool' by their peer group. And that probably wasn't of much interest to feminists.

The second difference is that teenagers, like the other groups mentioned back on pages 35–6, have fewer self-monitoring skills than mature adults. The parts of the brain we need to carry out 'executive functioning', which covers such things as self-discipline and long-term planning, are not fully formed until we're in our very late teens or early 20s. So it's hardly surprising that teenagers don't always do 'sensible'; or that a large proportion of younger teenagers smoke at some point in their adolescence. Even those who have been brought up to think sensibly and to respect their bodies are likely to have short phases when the need for immediate gratification, without too much thought of the consequences, is king.

So, feminists and others have used cigarette smoking in the past as a prop of rebellion, but without knowing its dangers. But youngsters now use the same behaviour to get the same effect, whilst knowing of the dangers, but ignoring them because they lack the mature skills to judge what they're doing and the risks that they're taking. It's highly unlikely that any other group of people would now take up smoking en masse to symbolise their retaliation against unreason!

Ultimately, as ever, it will only be those teenagers who have had all the 'right' programming who will go on to be fully addicted. But, sadly, there are so many young people around today whose upbringing has left them feeling rather inadequate and needy that there is a growth industry in addictive behaviour of all kinds. So, while older people are giving up smoking in greater numbers than ever, younger people are not only taking it up at least as much as ever, but also taking their smoking behaviour way beyond the teenage 'experimental' stage, and in greater numbers too.

Now that the dangers of smoking are so well understood, there is a sense in which one part, the 'innocent' part, of the history of smoking cigarettes is coming to an end. But it leaves a legacy that affects many of us. We are the inheritors of thousands of positive and memorable images associated with the smoking of cigarettes, which were foisted on to us by marketing people, advertisers and TV and film producers in those innocent earlier times. So far, those same persuaders have failed to work up equally powerful negative smoking stereotypes and the historic, pro-smoking stereotypes remain firm and unchallenged in our memories and in our culture. They're powerful enough to carry on generating positive images of smokers inside our heads, despite all the new thinking. After all, how many of us see Humphrey Bogart wielding a cigarette in *Casablanca* and think, 'What a saddo'?

Cigarettes in our private space

And that, by a curious twist, and with a following wind, takes us back to the inside of our heads. Where much of any cigarette gets smoked. Remember, this is the chapter of the book in which we're trying to discover why we choose cigarettes as our addictive substance, so now we can move on from the history of cigarettes and smoking (however eccentric) and start looking at the place cigarettes occupy, as objects, in both our inner and our outer 'space'.

Every one of us lives in two, quite different, worlds. And every one of us leads two, quite separate, lives. One of these lives we live privately, in an inner world, where we are heroes and heroines and act out our fantasies. It's in that world that we have affairs with film stars, pop stars or whoever, and tell ourselves stories about what we expect to happen next and how we expect ourselves to behave. Our other lives take place in the real, physical, solid, outside world where other people join us.

And, to all intents and purposes, our smoking of cigarettes takes place in two, quite separate, worlds, too. Each of which will affect our smoking behaviour slightly differently.

Cigarettes in the outside world

Let's take the way the real, solid, physical world affects us first, largely because it's an easier place to start. We may like to see ourselves as free spirits but our behaviour is still influenced in all sorts of ways by the outside world. It's affected by obvious things like laws, culture and peer pressure that we come up against on a daily basis and are usually aware of being affected by. But it's also affected, in ways we don't often think about, by the very existence of physical objects themselves. If you don't believe me, just think how our behaviour has been affected by the arrival in our lives of computers, or of mobile phones. Whatever did we do before them? How did we make contact with other human beings?

And what about those little white tubes themselves, cigarettes? What did we do before them and how does their existence affect our smoking behaviour?

There are a number of what might be called the basic 'givens' of why we should choose to use cigarettes as our addictive substance. Let's now take a look at them one by one.

- Cigarettes have to exist before we can want to smoke them.

I can't imagine that people used to roll up dock leaves and set light to them in ancient times. Did fourteenth-century man gasp, 'If only they would create something I could smoke!' We have to assume that any desire we might have to smoke cigarettes comes as a consequence of smoking's associations with nicotine and of the satisfaction we get from our ritual behaviour. It certainly doesn't arise as the result of a hard-wired human need to inhale containerised gases while wafting little sticks around in our fingers. That might sound a totally obvious and unnecessary thing to say, but it might just get you wondering about how you would cope if cigarettes simply didn't exist. Or if you simply didn't allow that they existed (now there's a thought!)

- We have to have the opportunity to smoke cigarettes.

True, smokers are very skilled at making room in their lives for the weed, but even hardened smokers might have problems making time or space if they were in a space shuttle (not that they'd be considered healthy enough to go up in one anyway), or out of doors in the Antarctic. What I really mean to emphasise here is that cigarettes and smoking come to smokers opportunistically. If you had never been offered that first one, what would you be doing about it now? There's no answer to that question, but again, it should keep in mind the idea that the opportunity for each cigarette that's going to be smoked has to *keep on* cropping up. You have to keep on making space for it. So opportunity does actually occupy a very important place in people's smoking behaviour. However, opportunity is not the same as availability. Though we might have access to cigarettes, and there might even, theoretically, be time for us to smoke them, if the opportunity to put a cigarette in the mouth and set light to it isn't there, then we just won't get around to doing it. For example what happens when someone's driving fast round a race track, having a hot shower (or a cold one for that matter), running a marathon, or sleeping? Do they start lighting up then?

Take opportunity away, and somehow desire goes with it. Could any of us genuinely say that having a cigarette would be at the forefront of our mind if we were driving at 100 mph round Brand's Hatch, or that we spend our sleeping time desperately craving a cigarette?

- Cigarette smoking has to be, by and large, acceptable to enough people.

We don't want to feel totally ostracised for doing it. Historically, as we've seen, smoking has even been encouraged so, for example, many, if not most, adults smoked around the time of the Second World War, when cigarettes were made freely available. However, if there was enough condemnation or mockery of cigarettes, in their own right, and if enough embarrassing punishments were dreamt up for the people who smoked them, then the great majority of smokers would give up. People have to feel that their personal benefit outweighs their personal cost and if it doesn't they will nearly always drop a behaviour. Would you still want to smoke if the cigarettes you smoked produced the smell of a fart, and if people in the street pelted you with rotten tomatoes every time you lit up?

- Nine-tenths of people have their first fag in response to peer pressure.

Fortunately many of them will not carry on with smoking behaviour much beyond an early, often teenage, stage. Which goes to prove that those who do carry on are not made to by the outside influence itself, otherwise everyone would go the same way. That aside, the underlying 'given' here is that most of us did not actively and independently want to have that first cigarette. It would have at least made some sense if we'd ended up addicted to ice cream.

Those four 'givens' are the most basic conditions that have to be met before we get to the point of seeing cigarettes as being our means to an end. But in addition to the givens there are many other, more variable, external pressures that will have influenced our decision to use cigarettes to meet our needs, and we'll come back to these soon. But before we do that, we'll take a look at the 'givens' of our other world, the one which only exists inside our own heads.

Cigarettes in our inside world

The inside of our heads is as real a space to us as the outside world. We live huge chunks of our lives in that space, day-dreaming, planning, talking to ourselves, and so on. And one of the most bizarre things about human behaviour is that we do things as much in reaction to what is going on inside our own heads as in reaction to what is going on outside. Many incentives and disincentives come from deep inside us. We're as likely to choose a particular perfume on the grounds that it reminds us of good times spent with a lover, as because it's being marketed prominently. And in spite of medical guidelines, we won't go running to doctors with unknown pains, if we keep hearing a beloved Granny's ghostly voice saying, 'No need to make a fuss, it's only a scratch.'

This inside world also has certain basic demands, which are as necessary as the 'givens' already described, before we start to see cigarettes as our means to an end. The first one is the equivalent of the 'given' in the external world that says that cigarettes actually have to exist before we can want to smoke them.

- We have to believe in cigarettes before we can want to smoke them.

It's pretty much the same situation as with ghosts. Before ghosts can scare us we have to believe in them and in their power to affect us negatively. Before cigarettes can attract us we have to believe in them and in their power to affect us positively. In other words, deep down, we have to think that a cigarette is more than just a collection of bits of shredded tobacco and paper sheets, we have to believe in it **as a force**.

- The smoking of cigarettes has to support the way we see ourselves.

We wouldn't keep a dog if we saw ourselves as a cat person, and we wouldn't elect to smoke a cigarette (even to get emotional needs met) if cigarettes didn't fit some kind of internal image of ourselves. Which means that when we light up we do it in ways that will reflect that inner image.

If John sees himself as a sociable chap, for example, he will have a cigarette because he understands that cigarettes are one of the acceptable props of the social settings that he likes, which might be a gathering of people, or a place like a wine bar or a club. And he will smoke a cigarette at a time when he thinks that smoking one is likely to be approved of, or at least not disapproved of, for example when having a drink, or after a meal, but definitely not in church. He will smoke when he thinks that having a cigarette will help him fit in, and make him feel that he's being properly social.

On the other hand, if Mike sees himself as in some way anti-social, and feels that he's an anti-society (with all its petty restrictions) person, he'll get his cigarettes out when it pleases him, without consideration for other people's feelings. He's as likely as not to smoke around someone he believes disapproves of cigarettes, or somewhere smoking is banned, because he will see both as 'getting back' at the world. And he will see the cigarette that he has used to do that as a prop in the hands of his little (inner) anti-social self.

In both of those cases our hero will feel some kind of inward approval of his behaviour; he will hear a little voice in his head that is giving him permission to smoke in those circumstances, and which will endorse what he already thinks of himself.

Those are the main basic 'givens' about the inner world of cigarettes. There are fewer than about the outer world, because there are fewer variables. And those that there are mostly boil down to those old coping skills and attitudes again. We will never (even if we have been introduced to cigarettes by a 'friend', and even during periods when smoking cigarettes is encouraged by the outer world) end up absolutely addicted to cigarettes if we do not have addictive thoughts and needs. Equally we will never, even if charismatic Humphrey Bogart was a smoker, and gorgeous Kate Moss is a smoker, use cigarettes to make ourselves attractive to the opposite sex, if inner voices keep on telling us we'll be disgusting if we smoke them.

Inner v. outer

If there is ever a tussle between the pressures of the inner and the outer worlds, with a smoker it's usually the inner world that wins, for good or ill. For example, a loyal Irish smoker might believe it wrong to light up in a public place today (given that new anti-smoking laws have just been passed). But if they remained loyal to their inner rebel (a characteristic that they had developed after a childhood full of messages that said never kow-tow to authority), they would have a dilemma on their hands. The outer world says, 'No cigarette!', but the inner world says, 'A cigarette is a necessary weapon in the war against tyranny.' Which wins?

The clincher will usually be that the addictive personality won't be able to face up to the inner conflict, and will turn to their addictive substance to manage the emotional turmoil. Meaning that the loyal

Irish smoker will end up saying, 'Oh, sod it,' and light up even though they no longer really fancy a fag!

Which really confirms that, in a non-dictatorial society, our inner world will always have greater power over us than our outer one.

Ultimately, though, it really doesn't matter which way round things work at the deepest levels. All that matters is that the solution to the problem of smoking cigarettes is simple. We need to establish what we want for ourselves in our lives today, and we need to understand what it was that had power over us in the past. With those two things in mind, we can come to some free and up-to-date decisions about which of those influences still have anything useful left to offer us. And then we can quit the primitive and impractical practice of smoking cigarettes.

External influences

We've just looked at a number of external and internal givens, that is, things that pretty much have to be in place for any smoker, both in the world and in their head, before they can see smoking cigarettes as a viable way of responding to their addictive neediness. Now we're going on to look at the rather more specific influences that may have affected any one of us personally. Either because they had individual relevance for us or because they were part of the wonderfully named *zeitgeist*, or spirit of the age.

I've gone to great lengths to push the idea that the greatest influences on our smoking behaviour happened way back in childhood, and before you read on it's hugely important that you remember to keep that idea at the forefront of your mind. The influences we're going on look at now are those that other people might believe to be the only ones of any consequence and you don't want to fall into that easy belief trap. You've wised up since beginning this book and I hope that as you go through the following pages, covering external influences, you will be able to see why they wouldn't have stood a chance of 'converting' you to smoking if you hadn't been programmed to 'give in' to them.

I could simply have drawn up lists of all the things that might influence any of us into choosing one behaviour over another. But as that seems a bit unfocused, I've decided to break things down into broad categories. And I'm going to start with one area of life, which we've only mentioned briefly so far, but that seems to me to be hugely significant. For most of the past it was thought of as just about the biggest influence of all on the way we lived our lives, but in the second part of the twentieth century its importance was questioned by some very loud voices. Say it quietly but we are finally allowed to speak of it; and as I've now introduced the controversial idea and it's too late to turn back, we're going to start by considering ...

The impact of gender on smoking behaviour

Men and women just aren't the same, thank goodness. And thank goodness we can say it again – life just becomes so much more interesting!

I'm going to deal with this section in two parts, one for each sex. It's important to read both parts, though, because although it's a convenience to say that one set of influences or behaviours belongs entirely to one sex: that's never going to be the whole story. That can only be a rule of thumb, and it's always going to be more important for us to discover what has affected us personally than to be rigid in our expectations. Anyway, it's terribly important to know all that we can about the other sex, especially now we're no longer forced to think that they're just like us (but possibly in denial).

I'm going to draw up lists of factors which are more likely to influence one sex than another, so that, as always, given the right pre-programming, a particular male or female might have been influenced by some combination of them into favouring cigarettes.

As a woman who doesn't want to show bias, I'm going to start with men, but no hierarchy's intended!

Testosterone

We might as well start with something that's already been referred to on a couple of occasions. And that is the hormone testosterone. This is the hormone that 'makes a man a man'. Because of his high levels of testosterone (women have testosterone, too, and the higher the level, the more male characteristics a woman has) a man is naturally aggressive, competitive and single-minded. All things being relative, including levels of testosterone, not all men will actually function like that, though some will. Most will show some of those characteristics some of the time.

How can all this affect a man's chances of smoking? Well, an aggressive feeling is going to become overwhelming if a man has no outlet for it and hasn't learnt how to deal with it in a harmless or healthy way. So if he has all the other pre-programming in place and then he gets swamped by feelings of aggression, he's likely to respond to the male stereotypes, do the 'macho' thing, and smoke. It's the 'red mist' factor, when testosterone fires up, inarticulacy reigns, thoughts and considerations of caution go out of the window and primitive gratifications are snatched.

High levels of competitiveness will affect chances of smoking as well. Especially in adolescence. After all, what young male wants to look weaker, softer, more cowardly, less cool, than his mates? And indifference to physical fearfulness is part of the age-old tradition of masculine toughness, isn't it? So, if a boy is brought up to believe that smoking equals hard, and he has a need to compete with the pack, then he's going to smoke.

The single-minded aspect of testosterone is a double-edged sword, ironically. It cuts both ways. If a high-testosterone chap decides that smoking is not for him, or that it was once but now he's giving up, then he's likely to stick with his decision, come hell or high water. But if he sees himself as a smoker, it's going to take a bomb to shift the idea.

Part of the reason for this is that high testosterone levels mean that men are less likely than women (though the difference is being offset by changes in women's social behaviour) to look at all the implications, all the knock-on consequences of their behaviour, such as unpopularity or heart failure. A woman is usually much more competent than a man at 'talking an idea through' internally while she assesses behavioural cause and effect. As in, 'I'm feeling really pissed off and everyone else is having a fag, which seems to make them feel better, but if I take this one cigarette that's being offered to me I might not be able to resist the next time, Dan might think I'm behaving like a slut, and anyway I hated that ad on the telly, the one which showed how that woman was dying of cancer but still kept on smoking and wiping the nasty, greasy stuff off her skirt, so I'd better not have it, because you never know.' Yes, chaps, it really does go like that. A man, on the other hand, is much more likely to say to himself, 'I'm pissed off, I know I shouldn't, but what the hell,' then go ahead and light up.

Smoking as a man's club

We saw from that magnificent poem earlier on that the start of the twentieth century was also the start of the smoking century for women. Some very 'fast', or very radical, women had smoked before that, but basically smoking was seen as a male sport. It had its own special tools and implements; its own uniform (for the upper classes at least, with their velvet smoking jackets and caps); its own rituals; and for long periods of history it came hand in glove with a Masonic secrecy that excluded women. They weren't allowed near the stuff, not if they were halfway respectable at least.

The shock waves from centuries of maleness are still felt. The 'club' culture that went with smoking in the past may often be shared with women now, but an association between male team sports and smoking remains strong, and every pub in the land with a large-screen TV is also a waiting room for the men's cancer ward. If a kid grows up in that kind of macho culture he's virtually growing up with a permission to smoke included in his inheritance.

Cultural stereotyping
The old cliché, but it holds true. From soldiers sitting patiently in dug-outs, to Humphrey Bogart in innumerable films, to Cold War spies, to Marlboro Man, the images of men who were 'real men', who fought bravely, treated women with ironic disdain, ran the world or rode the range all included cigarettes as part of the uniform. They've been very powerful images to shake off. For generations, boys have grown up wanting all the paraphernalia of their heroes, and if the loneliness, fear, heroics, or romantic moments of their heroes came accessorised with cigarettes, then that's how they wanted to kit themselves out, too.

Being my own boss
This attitude can really also be seen as a by-product of testosterone, but it does come with an anthem all of its own – Frank Sinatra's *My Way*. These are men who find it difficult working in a team, men who can't stand being forced into nine-to-five routines, men who love the idea of the open road, and men who have a dream, but what they all share is a dislike of being controlled. Of course, there are women who feel the same way, but men outnumber them vastly. And their constant refrain goes along the lines of, 'Nobody tells me what to do,' which may be fine if their basic ideas are good ones, but won't help them much if they're wanting to do things that are doomed to failure. If a man who feels like this sees smoking as part of an overall rejection of domination by others, then he's more likely to smoke than not. The flip side is that he may decide to take a stand against smoking if he's in a culture that embraces it.

Association with work and colleagues
Traditional working environments such as factories and heavy industry have a much higher proportion of smokers than workplaces associated

with white-collar workers. And as they also tend to employ more men than women, it follows that working-class men smoke more than average. Explanations given for these high levels of smoking include the suggestion that the work is often repetitive and may feel unrewarding. But these aren't reasons for smoking, they're only reasons for feeling bored. And why should smoking be a panacea for boredom? Realistically, a large part of the problem seems to come down to the sense that smoking has historically been part of an industrial lifestyle, and that many working men, being by and large traditionalists, still feel a kind of loyalty to the smoking behaviour. For them to give up would feel like a betrayal of a long-standing working culture and of the mates who are in it with them.

Another, often basically younger, group of men who are employed in what they see as 'high intensity' jobs, often associate smoking with their work, as well. Their work is high-pressure, perhaps commission-based, often target-led, such as sales, and it comes with a perceived need for safety valves. It's almost as if men in these jobs see their status as dependent on the number of safety valves they have to open to release all their pent-up tension. As though their self-image relies on their being able to 'cope well' with pressure. Because cigarettes will provide the most conspicuous and high-profile safety valves, the more that are smoked, the more evident the man's furious commitment to the work. And, again, the more that are smoked, the greater his commitment to his mates if they're smoking, too. Having a cigarette together may demonstrate a kind of bonding for men who aren't good at showing camaraderie in other ways.

Sports
It's ironic but smoking does seem to be associated with some, mainly masculine, sports. Darts, snooker and motor racing, for example, not to mention football, still have a smoky image. It's not that the players are necessarily smokers these days, more that either the supporters are, or that cigarettes and smoke are part of the scenery of the sports. Darts and snooker matches still look as though they're being held in a dark fug, and until very recently cigarette logos were part of the uniform of motor racing. And although there are lots of women fans of these sports, the generally masculine atmosphere hasn't changed much since the 60s and 70s. Times when smoking was still thought of as 'tough' or devil-may-care. It's down to image again really, but consciously or not, some men still seem to associate themselves with the old values.

Manual labour

This is tongue in cheek, but knowing what to do with their hands is a problem for a lot of men. No man likes to look pointless, and it's easy to look pointless if you've got nothing to carry in your hands, or nothing to do with your hands when you're sitting down. A cigarette fulfils two basic functions here: firstly it gives a man something to carry, and secondly it gives him something to do. It will fulfil a similar purpose for a woman, but a man's hand movements when smoking are different from a woman's. They're harder and more 'purposeful', which throws up the intriguing possibility that what men are really wanting to do all along as they smoke is to be constructive. Men are hard-wired for tool use, in a way that women aren't, so maybe for men smoking cigarettes is just a way of fobbing off a deep-seated desire to be crafting something.

That's not been an exhaustive list but, hopefully, some part of it should gel for you if you're a man. Or if it doesn't, the suggestions should, at least, prompt you into thinking about whether there was some other, predominantly masculine, factor that influenced the choice you made to smoke cigarettes as a way of supplying your emotional needs.

Because knowing what has influenced our decision to smoke means having ammunition in our fight back against it.

Girls' turn, now.

Oestrogen and cortisol

Just as testosterone is the mainly male hormone, oestrogen is the mainly female one, but cortisol, also, has a part to play in women's behaviour. High levels of the hormone cortisol produce anxiety and worry, which are emotions felt by many people who smoke. It just so happens that women have naturally higher levels of this hormone in their bodies.

Oestrogen is the hormone that most women are more familiar with. It's the one associated with periods and all the mood swings that take place during the menstrual cycle. One phase of those mood swings is usually a combination of depression and irritability, which means women have a very short fuse at certain times of the month. If you add a very short temper to all the pre-programmed neediness of addictive people (which we've talked of before in some detail), then you can see how snatching up a cigarette might seem like a good idea to a woman under stress. The nicotine in the cigarette will give a quick burst of a chemical that will counteract the depression and irritability, and although the effect of that will only last for a very brief length of time, her short-term thinking will ignore any longer-term implications. Especially as one of the other well-known effects around the time of a woman's period is the female refrain, 'Don't even **think** of trying to tell me what to do!', which she's every bit as likely to yell at her own 'inner authority' as at her long-suffering bloke!

Cortisol affects both men and women, but the naturally higher levels in women mean that they are usually more likely than men to choose to escape from unpleasant situations rather than to confront them ('time of the month' notwithstanding). And if they can't escape those situations for some reason, their anxiety levels will be quite high. This means that a lot of women are 'worry smokers', believing that the cigarettes they smoke will help to calm them down, allowing them to deal with the stresses caused by those confrontations. However, this is only a short-term effect, as we've seen.

There is another hormonal cause of female worry. Oestrogen opens up pathways and language centres in the brain that are usually helpful in making women flexible. But this effect can go into overdrive and sometimes women, when faced with decision-making situations, can see too many options, too many alternative ways of doing something, or too many ways something might go wrong. Little voices in their heads overdo the multi-tasking thing and leave them scrambling to find certainties and fixed points. If they can't find any reassuring ones, then ciggies can seem to offer a reliable alternative! Of course, we all know that there is just one certain outcome cigarettes can be relied on to provide: poorer health.

Stress

In a way this brings us on to stress. Stress affects men as well as women, but until fairly recently it was less likely that men would 'own up' to it. Women, on the other hand, occasionally seem to define themselves by how much they suffer. Stress isn't something that only exists in the mind and it does have physical consequences, but it can be the case that we create it for ourselves: we can increase the stress we experience through the attitudes we have to events. These days, women are sometimes encouraged to see as stressful things and events that in the past would have been seen as natural, or inevitable; things like pregnancy and childbirth, bringing up children, death of parents and long working hours. In the past, women might have thought of all these as hard work, but not necessarily as 'stressful', a word that suggests 'too hard to be reasonable'. If a woman is pre-programmed to feel needy and resentful, then sees her life as being too hard to be reasonable, what response could feel more reasonable than having a cigarette?

None of which should be read as suggesting that women's lives are easy-peasy. Women are now feeling the need to take on roles that mean they have to work incredibly long hours just to fit everything in and get everything done. If they are to be as perfect as the stereotypes that they are working to, that is.

Female stereotyping

Male stereotypes in the past tended to be made up of hard men; and men could have failings in all sorts of departments, as long as they remained hard. But female stereotypes tended to demand perfection of one sort or another from women. And they still do, even though today's style of perfection is different from yesterday's. Early- to mid-twentieth-century images of femininity meant that women felt they should try to live up to the glamour of style legends such as Marlene Dietrich or Audrey Hepburn, both of whom were famously portrayed as smokers. What young woman hasn't looked with envy at that gloriously iconic poster of Audrey Hepburn in *Breakfast at Tiffany's* in which she smiles seductively whilst elegantly holding an immense cigarette holder in the air? But in the same century other images expected women to be homemakers and bread-bakers, people who kept the home fires burning till the gallant boys came home. The two stereotypes were opposites that it was impossible to reconcile. A woman could be desirable (and smoke); or she could be subservient to a gallant (and smoking) male. Either way, cigarettes came as part of the package and with an endorsement that whichever sex you were, they gave you some kind of power over the other sex.

When feminism really kicked in in the 1960s, it provided those women who weren't already smoking with yet more incentives to take up the habit. If a woman was going to be as good as a man – if not better, in fact – then she would have to do even more of what men did, and two of the things that men did were behave as sexual predators and smoke. A new female stereotype emerged, one that showed women as being sexually and behaviourally equal with men. As sexuality was in any case linked to smoking, a woman who wanted to be both equal and sexy had a double incentive to smoke. She would look like someone who could take the sexual initiative *and* she could buy her own cigarettes for afterwards.

Ladette culture

This is really only the making of a new stereotype. From being convinced in the 1960s and '70s that the way forward was for women to become confident that they could be as good as men, some girls have gone to the extreme of wanting to be *more* blokey than the average bloke – 'Anything you can do I can do better, but with knobs on'. And that has meant pushing their bodies to take on board just about every toxic substance, provided they take it to excess, simply to prove that they can. Which of course they can't, really, at least not for any length of time. And neither could any man, if the intake was pro rata, pound for pound of body weight. Ladette behaviour has been a very dangerous development for girls, it's led to binge drinking and binge smoking of industrial quantities of chemicals that in the past could only have been tolerated by total lushes. Smoking and drinking on such a scale is going to be harmful enough to the long-term health of even those young women who know when they're overdoing things, but believe that they should be able to 'take it' for a while. How much worse will the effect be on someone who is less in control, who's already got addictive needs in place? How easy will it be for a desperately inadequate girl, who has to boost her ego somehow, to acknowledge that she's constantly taking on more than she can cope with?

Appearance

One thing that feminism didn't affect, except in the case of a very few hard-liners, was women's obsession with how they look. Especially their obsession with how they look in terms of body shape. And something that nearly all women smokers believe with an almost religious fervour, despite the evidence of porky, chain-smoking darts players, is that cigarettes keep you thin. Cigarettes don't keep you thin, of course, except when they are used to replace healthy nourishment – and then it's the smokers who are starving themselves, the cigarettes themselves are doing nothing. What keeps this idea going is that when an addictive person gives up one substance, that is, cigarettes, they're more likely to replace it with another, such as fattening biscuits or chocolate and so quitting smoking becomes associated with weight gain. Which is actually a rather different scenario.

So, for women, smoking becomes attractive by its association with slimness and with the richer, more exotic, more successful lifestyles that tend to go with being slim. Most women aren't daft enough to believe that smoking cigarettes actually leads directly to success, except, presumably, for tobacco barons, but they do subconsciously link the behaviour with certain kinds of success. And some of the most attractive and alluring forms of success in women's eyes are those that are connected to the world of beauty and modelling. Even *Absolutely Fabulous,* the absolutely brilliant TV send-up, hasn't cured some women of their addiction to that perceived world of 'glamour'. It doesn't matter that smoking leads to cancer and strokes, or that it ruins the skin, or that most women will never get anywhere near such lifestyles, the connection between cigarettes, stick-thin models and big fat wallets is just too strong to ignore.

Looking and feeling the part

For women, as for men, hands and cigarettes go together. But there does seem to be a gender gap in the way this connection is made. Women make more open gestures with their cigarettes than men do. They also hold cigarettes differently. Men can be seen pointing with their cigarettes, holding them like darts, or cradling them in their palms, but women more usually hold their cigarettes between their first two fingers, hold them slightly out and away from their bodies and make less pointed movements with them.

Women place cigarettes into their mouths more slowly and carefully, and then draw them away from their lips more slowly, rather as if they were using cigarettes as an extension of what they were saying. Perhaps some women smoke because they feel they're not able to express their thoughts adequately without adding physical or visual support to what they've got to say? That really shouldn't be taken too seriously, it's only a thought but, joking aside, the use of touch and gesture in women's smoking behaviour does form quite a serious part of the pleasure they get from it. If all the ritual of lighting up and of touching and holding a cigarette were divorced from the smoking of it, the pleasure in smoking that women would lose would probably be greater than the pleasure lost by men. Overall, women seem to need something to *touch* with their hands where men need something to *do* with their hands.

Vive la différence

Looking at all the above, it seems that many of the external influences on men's smoking are connected to their historic relationship with the world of work and daily activity, and may also come out of a sort of awareness of class or politics, or a combination of the two. The external influences on women, on the other hand, seem to be rather different.

They seem to be more connected with gender relationships and concerns, and with a consciousness of appearance and acceptability. But if a generalisation like that makes you mad and gets you saying, 'No, no, that's so sexist. It's all down to ...', so much the better, because it's stimulated you to decide what has affected you. And at least half the purpose of this book is to make you aware of *why* you smoke, while the other half (which we're just reaching) is to make you challenge those reasons and finally give up the behaviour.

Whatever happened in the past and whatever the specific influences that may have affected any one of us individually, something is happening now which is going to affect thousands, if not hundreds of thousands of people. And, whether or not it sounds sexist to say it, women are the ones who are in the firing line.

An alarming development is taking place. It's alarming in its own right, and it's alarming for the future. Not only is the highest percentage of smokers in any age group to be found amongst 20- to 24-year-olds, but, for the first time in history, it's young women who are starting to smoke in greater numbers than young men. Among 16- to 19-year-olds, the figures are 28 per cent compared with 22 per cent, and the disparity will get worse as more boys than girls are now giving up smoking. So, although male smokers still outnumber female ones over the age of 25, there can only be one direction for this new trend and that is towards worse and worse health for women. This conclusion is supported by all the research, which shows that women are now having strokes and heart attacks in dramatically increasing numbers. But, ultimately they won't be the only ones who will suffer.

Men, women ... and children

There are bound to be many, multi-layered causes behind the upward trend in smoking, some of which we've already covered in what's been said in this book. However, rather than spend pointless years investigating which of them are most to blame, why don't we just get stuck straight in and make the smoking of cigarettes by anyone, male or female, seem more and more absurd, and less and less acceptable. While we're at it, we should start by making it completely unacceptable amongst pregnant women, because they are responsible not only for the immediate health of their own lives, but also for the health of their babies, *and for the long-term health of the next generation.*

This is vital. Consider the following facts about how mothers affect their children's health:

- Smoking cigarettes will affect a woman's ability to carry a baby at all. Smokers are less physically fit than other women and are more likely to be ill during pregnancy and to have miscarriages.

- In the womb, the baby's development will be affected by exposure to the chemicals in cigarettes – smokers' children are smaller, more sickly, likely to be mentally slower, and much more likely to be difficult babies to look after.

- Smoking affects the way mothers deal with their babies. We know that smokers are more likely to be anxious people, showing emotionally needy behaviour themselves (partly down to their own backgrounds, but also down to their addiction to roller-coaster toxins). This will make them behave in ways that are unsettling around their children. And that, in turn, will lead to their own children being more at risk of developing dependent personalities, and so to becoming addicts of one sort or another (not only to becoming addicts of tobacco).

- Exposing a child to passive smoking will increase their risk of developing many illnesses in later life, specifically childhood asthma and, it is now believed, lung cancer.

- Mothers are role models for the next generation, not only for their own children, but for all children who come into contact with them. If you set the example of smoking to children around you – well, you know the rest.

We may not like to confront any of that, and we may not like being dictated to. But who has the right to leave the next generation to confront it all, and who has the right to dictate that a child's health should suffer, just so that we can have our immediate needs met? All of us, but most especially mothers, will feel so much happier knowing that by stopping smoking we've not only beaten our own addiction, but also met the needs of those people who matter most to us.

Pro-smoking influences

Now let's take a look at more of the external factors that may influence our decision to smoke. The first of these continues neatly from the previous section. However, it is not gender-dependent as such and neither are the ones that follow. Most of them are matters that will affect both sexes more or less equally.

Parents' habits

This is much more straightforward than all that stuff in previous chapters about inner coping skills and attitudes. Here we are simply covering the question of whether or not our parents (or one of them) ever smoked. We're all much more likely to do something our parents have done than not, from playing the piano to gardening, overeating and having violent arguments. This is so even if, as part of the inevitable teenage disgust with parents, an adolescent child of smoking parents rejects the whole idea of smoking as repulsive – they still remain much more at risk of smoking at some later stage in their lives than a child of non-smoking parents. And, despite what I said above, there is actually a slight gender consideration here, inasmuch as, if it's only the mother of the family who smokes, any daughter she has is more likely to identify with and copy her behaviour than any son she has. The same pretty obviously applies the other way around, with fathers and sons. A girl usually wants to be like Mummy, a boy wants to be like Daddy.

Inevitably, there are other factors that will affect the chances of the children of smokers smoking themselves. These include the levels of respect they feel towards their parents, and the question of whether or not peer or cultural pressures (i.e., friends' attitudes, or TV, film and magazine images) will push them more firmly away from smoking than their identification with their parents is pushing them towards it. But the bottom line for most of us is that what we see our parents doing becomes our norm, and it will always be easier for us to accept it than to reject it. And it doesn't affect things one jot if our parents give up cigarettes at some stage whilst we're growing up: the damage will already have been done.

So: completely non-smoking parents produce more non-smoking children than smoking parents. It's that simple.

Class

What I'm about to say may be considered to be a very 1960s, black-and-white, kitchen-sink drama sort of effect, that is if there isn't actually a taboo on mentioning it at all, but health care professionals know this to be absolutely true: statistically, someone from the working, or manual, classes is at least *twice as likely* to smoke as someone from the higher social classes. And when we come to people who sleep rough and people who are generally dispossessed, the rate of smoking runs at about *90 per cent*. Premature deaths from lung cancer are *five times higher* for unskilled workers than for professional men, and poorer smokers smoke cigarettes more intensively, drawing nicotine more deeply into their lungs, than wealthier ones. So it seems that, at least as far as smoking goes, class is still with us.

Comments that appear to suggest that smoking is okay for people from the lower classes, 'because it's the only pleasure they have', only serve to complicate things. Why would anyone want to teach people that harming their health is a class right? It's also rather insulting for those working class people (still just about in the majority) who manage their lives perfectly well without cigarettes.

There is some evidence that it is the children of the middle class and higher social groups who find it most easy to quit smoking after taking it up. So it appears that attitudes to self-management are involved, with the middle – or, if you like, the managing – classes being more likely to be self-starters and to believe in self-help than those who come from classes with a long history of being on the receiving end of management. And there is probably another effect at work here, which is that the children of manual workers will see more of their families smoking well into middle age with fewer people around them setting the example of giving up smoking. If smoking behaviour becomes associated with our own class and our own 'group', we are much more likely to show solidarity with the behaviour and to identify with the effects of the behaviour, however undesirable they are. A child of poorer parents may actually come to believe that it is part of their 'birthright' to feel a bit ill as they get older. It may become an unspoken expectation that if Uncle John coughs and has chest pains after years of smoking, that's pretty much what's going to come to us, like inheriting his curly hair, or Granny's tea set.

That is if there is no challenge to the expectation. But every poorer smoker who gives up cigarettes is breaking that mould and they're helping to change the future for someone else as well.

Mental health

I mentioned drug addicts, alcoholics and schizophrenics near the start of the book as being all more likely to smoke than the general population; then in The Big Birds of Influence I said autism was also a risk factor for smoking. As autism is a mental development disorder that affects the ability to relate and to think about oneself from the outside, and addiction and schizophrenia are mental health issues, there might not seem to be an obvious connection, but all these problems do have similar implications for smoking behaviour.

All mental disorders lead to different ways of thinking. And any difficulties we have with controlling our thoughts, or with judging how our thoughts might affect what we do and so our health or safety, put us more at risk of addictive behaviour generally and, inevitably, of smoking. That probably sounds a bit daft, as alcoholism and drug addiction are already addictions anyway. But having an addiction of any sort puts the addict at greater risk of developing another kind of addiction.

Remember, I said earlier that if an alcoholic or drug addict gives up their primary addiction but then carries on smoking, they're much more likely to relapse. That is because they haven't worked out and dealt with the original addictive thoughts. Unfortunately it's the same with all these cases, and with similar mental problems such as depression and bipolar disorder (manic depression). They all affect a person's ability to think a situation through calmly and healthily, and they also affect self-control. The consequence is that overall rates of addiction to smoking amongst people with mental health problems are at about 75 per cent, the highest overall rate of any group.

Apart from people with schizophrenia, which research seems to suggest is affected in unusual ways by nicotine, people with most mental health and development disorders will nearly always be helped by stopping smoking. We all, wherever we're coming from, need the maximum possible basic physical fitness to recover from any health problem. We also all have a deep-seated need to regain or develop the best possible control over our lives so that we can feel as good as possible about ourselves. Imagine how much more people will benefit from increased levels of fitness, and all that extra oxygen, when the problems they've had have included organising their thoughts and managing their emotions. For them it's going to be a win-win situation, squared.

The arts
This section is really more to do with image than with artistic endeavour itself. Smoking and the arts have often been associated and the association has been more than encouraged by films and books over the years. But sculptures and paintings don't exactly demand a creator who smokes, after all Michaelangelo managed to get by without. And Shakespeare wasn't famous for puffing on cigars as he wrote his sonnets and plays. Whatever myths advertisers and image-conscious artists might have liked to put about from time to time, creativity really isn't constipated by a lack of access to tobacco.

Maybe any genuine connection between the arts and smoking that has grown up over the years has had more to do with some of the unusual living arrangements and working hours of artists. Perhaps it has especially been to do with the loneliness and the lack of normal structure in the lives of creative artists, people who are often 'alternative' thinkers in the first place. And maybe the connection is also to do with the pendulum swing felt by people who work in the performing arts or in the world of exhibiting, for whom life is a series of pressured highs and tedious lows. But none of these effects actually demands a specific response or behaviour from anyone. Each of us is free to deal with any situation according to how we feel about it and about ourselves. There are still thousands of artists and performers around who don't need cigarettes as part of their lifestyle.

It is a fact, though, that musicians, painters and writers often see smoking as part of the job description – not as a way to overcome the monotony of the work, or as part of the camaraderie, but as part of the working practice itself. Whether that means seeing a cigarette slotted into the strings of a guitar as part of a youthful dream of fame, or seeing an over flowing ashtray next to an old Remington portable as part of the romance of writing, this toxic tool of the trade seems to have become a fixed symbol for creativity in some people's minds. And perhaps, without realising it, some artists expect it of themselves and then try very hard to live up to their own expectations.

If that is the case, as creative and free thinkers, perhaps artists should now work on becoming free of what is, after all, just a boring old stereotype. And perhaps they should try the effect of a boost of oxygen on their creativity at the same time.

Ritual

Is this an external factor? I think it quite probably is.

For a lot of people who've quit smoking, the thing that they find they miss the most is not the nicotine, or even the oral stimulation of having a cigarette in their mouth: it's the ritual activity they've always associated with smoking. And that effect is probably doubled for smokers who've been used to rolling their own.

Human beings love ritual, both for its own sake and, if it's shared with others, for the sense it brings of belonging to an exclusive club. We only have to think of societies like the Masons and of the delight that children get from things like passwords and shared secret codes to recognise the basic attraction. Smokers get rewards from both sources.

Let's look at the ritual first. There's all that business that we covered in the questionnaires of playing with the paraphernalia of smoking, of flicking lighters, tapping boxes (remember when cigarettes were tapped on silver cases?), rolling up little balls of paper and playing with them, etc. Then there's the lighting-up ritual itself. It may be less exciting now than in the days when real men lit matches on their thumbnails, but, all the same, the way a smoker lights up is usually very dear to their hearts (which makes that a really good target for change during the quitting process). There's often a tidying-up ritual involved, too, so all in all smoking a cigarette can provide smokers with a lot of time-consuming ritual activity, which also takes up their attention and allows them to escape from having to think about weightier matters.

Secondly, there's the reward smokers get from knowing that, in a general way, other smokers will be doing much the same sort of thing as themselves. That is, enjoying their smoke and separating themselves from the rest of life. Such shared behaviour, which nowadays is often carried out in a slightly furtive or self conscious way, gives them not only a shared experience but also a mutual understanding. And aren't we all looking for that?

Overall, smoking can seem to provide someone with a lot of little behaviours that will gratify their need for ritual, belonging and security. It's such a pity that it comes at such a price. And that it's so divisive, because what most smokers really need deep down is to find themselves acceptable.

X-factors

I'm now going to include some external factors that could be seen as not really belonging. This is because they are part and parcel of what happens to us individually. However, as they are often quoted as reasons (read excuses) for smoking, I will lump them in with the rest and you can decide for yourself whether or not you could ever think of them as having been influential.

Foreign travel
This is often given as the reason someone started smoking. It is certainly likely to be thought of as such, since so many people have had their first experience of 'abroad' during adolescence (a particularly vulnerable time), when they've travelled to countries where smoking has been taken much more for granted across a wide range of classes, ages etc. and where it is still sometimes seen as a fairly normal or acceptable part

of sophisticated behaviour. Many youngsters doing a student exchange have felt that smoking Gitanes, or similar, was part of the whole 'cultural experience' and then, having started it on holiday, have carried on with the smoking behaviour when they've got back home. But, equally many youngsters won't have started smoking when abroad, however many of the locals were smoking around them, and many of the locals won't have been smoking, either; so why blame another country or culture for our personal behaviour? The usual rules apply: an essential neediness has to be in place before someone can think that smoking cigarettes is an appropriate thing to do, whatever the circumstances.

Death

This is a hard one, especially when a close relative is involved. Sometimes death does just seem a stress too far, even for someone who might have lots of emotional coping skills in place under normal circumstances. People can often feel that nothing particularly matters any more after a death; or they can feel so dissociated from their usual selves and their normal responses that they end up copying things they have seen other people doing (in real life, or in films), which they see as being typical behaviours in the circumstances they now find themselves in. It's almost as if, when traumatised, we can think that a response like smoking is to be expected of us. But, as usual, even under these extreme circumstances we will find other people reacting differently, and even if we do start smoking as part of a reaction to trauma, we will only carry it on if we haven't learnt how to manage such complex feelings properly.

Major events

When people go through wars, natural catastrophes, accidents and other life-threatening or life-changing events, they be affected in exactly the same way as they are by the death of someone close. Shock and a sense of the world turning upside down can leave any of us feeling that all normal bets are off. But, as with death, if someone does start smoking at a time like this, they must already have an inappropriate set of thought processes in place for them to think that carrying on is preferable to returning to a healthier way of coping (see my comments on the Second World War and the general culture and acceptance of smoking on page 57).

And your excuse is...?

There are probably two main types of reaction that you could have had to all these various suggestions about which external factors may have affected your decision to smoke. One sort of reaction may have gone along the lines of, 'Oh, yes, I saw *Breakfast at Tiffany's* when I was 15 and I can remember thinking just how sexy and sophisticated Audrey Hepburn was. However silly it seems now, when I started smoking I know that some part of me wanted to be just like her. I even used to hold my cigarette the same way,'

Or, you may have thought something along the lines of, 'I never felt the need to smoke until my wife left me and then I thought, "Oh to hell with it. Other people smoke at times like this, why shouldn't I? I've got nothing else."'

A reaction such as either of these would tell you that you can now see how external forces will have worked on the emotional needs you already had in place from childhood. In the first example given above, those dominating needs would have been to be desirable like Audrey Hepburn, rather than remaining like your (unlovely?) self. And in the second, to have a relationship that defined who you are and made your life worth living (because you're nobody on your own?).

What the external forces have said to you is that cigarettes can be a form of salvation or solution to your, existing, problems. Which, of course, they can't be – they only make things worse. External forces simply operate as dishonest messengers, but, idiots that we are, we listen to them if we can't find answers to our own problems inside ourselves. Understanding the connections between all these things takes us at least halfway to breaking them and changing the behaviour. And that means at least halfway to stopping smoking.

But, on the other hand, your reaction to the suggestions about outside forces may have been more like, 'No, no, I wasn't particularly affected by any of those things there. In fact I don't believe that I've been affected by anything very much. I just like the taste of cigarettes,'

Which would be a bit disappointing, as that would sound as if you were falling back on an age-old defensive coping mechanism, like denial. But even if you haven't quite managed to recognise which externals had their effect on you yet, it's not too late. Go back over the last few pages to give yourself another chance either to find something you'd overlooked, or to use my list of externals to kick-start your own ideas and find some alternatives of your own (because you're most probably someone who prefers to do their own thing).

Even if you have already decided what things you think have affected you, it's still a useful exercise to do a written inventory of how many of them apply. Maybe you'll think of some more as you're doing it, anyway.

So, before we move on any further, make a list of any of the influences mentioned there which you think have, or even *may* have, affected your decision to start smoking cigarettes and to carry on doing so, beyond the point where you have found it possible to stop. If it's a person, don't spare them from having the finger pointed at them, however close they may have been to you, on the grounds that they weren't to know you'd copy them, or that they're lovely and you don't want to accuse them or to think badly of them. And don't overlook the possibility that a particular situation may have been influential in the choice you made, because, 'It's hardly surprising if I smoked then, it would have been hard not to'. We're not here to attack anyone else, or to criticise your own lack of strength. All that we're doing is trying to establish cause and effect. Knowledge is power.

Check, check and check again

You'll have noticed that I've asked you several times to go back over something and to write down what you've found out about your background or behaviour. At various stages of the book I've asked you to do a quick resumé of what you've discovered about yourself, or to write an inventory of the various forces that you think have affected your attitudes and behaviours. The idea behind doing all this work is that repetition is vital to learning, and writing things down is vital to remembering (especially when we get past the age of about six!), so going back over things helps us to establish them firmly in our minds. Hopefully, going through all those exercises has been useful in reminding you of where we are now and how we got here, and is also helping you to keep a tight hold of all the different strands we've covered, because we've come a long way from our starting point.

We're at the halfway stage now, and very soon we're going to twist those various strands into one strong link. In the first half of the book we concentrated on why you started, and have subsequently carried on with, your smoking behaviour. The second part is going to focus on stopping smoking and on what you're going to do afterwards to keep it up and to prevent relapses. You'll discover how to substitute healthy new behaviours for unhealthy old ones, and how to get clean, healthy satisfaction from life, instead of fuggy and unhealthy gratification, as you got in your smoky past.

But before we shift the focus, it's vital to do one more, yet bigger, resumé. We've covered the trigger feeling, we've had the trigger moment, and now it's time to get to the critical moment itself, the one when we actually light up.

We're going to focus on that moment, learn all about it, and then use it to turn you from being a 'person who smokes' into a person who 'used to smoke', but is now a *person who doesn't smoke!*

Going Critical
Or, From the trigger moment to the critical moment of choice

This is the moment when all our past comes into collision with the present and we decide to take one road into our future, rather than another.

If you think about it carefully, it's actually the only moment that really counts in your smoking life, because it's the moment when you make that decision to light up. It's the moment that takes you from simply being a needy, rebellious, anxious (or whatever) person, one who is in a particular set of circumstances, and turns you into a person who smokes.

I think that the best (and possibly most fun) way to do this next resumé will be to create a cartoon history of the things you've covered and discovered so far. Unless you're a pro, or have a lot of time on your hands, the easiest way to do this is probably using 'matchstick men' drawings.

I expect that most of us know the saying 'a picture is worth a thousand words', and that applies a thousand times more to drawing pictures of your own story. Each picture you draw should speak volumes about you and should help you to make better and better sense of yourself. And, with any luck, doing this exercise should be entertaining at the same time.

You'll need paper, pencils and crayons, or felt tips, and scraps of various sorts of materials.

How you started

The general idea is to get a visual impression down on paper of how your story looks so far, from childhood to the present day. So take a big sheet of paper (A3 at least) and start drawing at the far left, at the point when you're a baby. Do a little sketch of a pram or a cot to symbolise where you are, then draw in all those big birds, which were circling round above you at the time. You can add any little embellishments to them that you like, including drawing labels beside them and writing inside them what the birds' droppings consisted of. Go the whole hog if you want and make a collage instead, and stick bits and pieces on to your picture. Choose them to represent feelings you had and messages you received; lovely, soft, fluffy things, strokable velvet, scraps of glittery feathers, bits of rubbish, even real fag ends. Anything that you think got dropped down on to you from above. Think hard, be creative, and have fun.

As your story develops, draw yourself first as a little matchstick toddler who's learning how to crawl and play, and then make that child bigger and bigger, show it perhaps riding its bike, or playing with its toys, and add a little rucksack on to its back. That rucksack is very important because it is going to represent what the child is starting to carry with it, what we often call 'baggage' nowadays.

With each spurt of growth for the child you can take away a few of the birds, if you like, but add something to the rucksack, because the package of attitudes, and ideas about itself, that a child carries with it grows bigger and heavier all the time. The contents of those rucksacks are what set off the familiar 'trigger feeling', (which, once we've come to recognise it, we can start to call the Danger Alarm Bell) when, in the first place the child, then later the adult, comes across challenges to its coping abilities.

You need to show what's in the rucksacks, so have some fun making up little, personal parcels, like little wrapped Christmas presents, and stick on to them tiny labels describing the contents. The contents should be made up of the various attitudes to yourself and life that you described earlier on in the book, the ones that you've already decided led to your trigger feelings. Make up little parcels, marked with words like 'Anger', or with phrases like 'It's not fair!', or with whatever you feel belongs to you, and glue them on to your rucksack.

The next features you should add to your cartoon are little bits of the background detail of your story. These should include *places* where you will have been influenced by other people (such as school, clubs, France, where you did an exchange, etc.) Then add some props, like magazines, little TV sets and similar, which are to stand for *things* that you know affected your thinking over the years. Now add a few other little matchstick *characters*, to represent the people who have been influential in your life. They can be people you've known directly, or even people you've known indirectly, say through the media, so long as they have been style icons to you, or people whose ideas or behaviour you wanted either to copy or to reject. But they must have had some effect on your smoking behaviour. And then stick tiny little cigarettes in the hands or mouths of any people whose own smoking behaviour you think you might have copied.

As you are now

Now having created visuals of all the pre-programming that went into the making of the smoking behaviour of your little matchstick self, you can finally draw the latest version of you. You, as you are today. If you feel it's appropriate, make this version a bit bigger, and add details that you think define you as you are now: carrying a laptop or designer clothes bags, talking into your mobile, feeding a baby, whatever, but make the picture the image of the self whose smoking behaviour you want to challenge. You will still be carrying a rucksack on your back though (a bit battered by now) and stick on to it little parcels that stand for the final package of attitudes which you're also still carrying into your smoking behaviour every time you light up.

The trigger moment

You've drawn everything to do with yourself now, so what you're going to add in next is the trigger moment. It's time to look back at what you've said about the ingredients that are needed for one to 'happen'. You've got your trigger feelings lined up already in your rucksack. So when you've checked what's needed, scatter the rest of the ingredients around that latest version of yourself, drawing in the location as background, the people as other matchstick drawings, etc. Then put in some tiny detailing to represent any sensory ingredients that form part of your trigger moment. Perhaps a grape seed to stand in for the smell of wine, or a few crotchets to suggest a sentimental tune? Then finish this section off with some written words that describe the emotional circumstances of a typically 'overwhelming' trigger moment.

As you stand back to admire your handiwork, you should be looking at a very graphic chart of how you get yourself to the all-important stage of feeling you **need** a cigarette. When you look at it like this, it should be easy (if you've done a great job) to see that it's got more to do with what's going on inside you than what's going on outside you. That, in truth, *smoking really is all in the mind.*

The critical moment of choice

As far as you possibly can put yourself into that very particular frame of mind right now, as you're looking at your own picture, and tap into all the sensory experience you've symbolised there as well. Remind yourself of just how different parts of your body feel when you feel you can no longer go without a cigarette. And remember, for some people that feeling may only come once in a month, for others it may come every ten minutes. There are no hard and fast rules about this side of it, it's only to do with the intensity of the experience. Go through the physical sensations you have at a time like this, from head to foot, in minute detail. Pay particular attention to the inside places: check any tension in your head; check the sensations down through the core of your body, in your tummy, in your lungs – what's your breathing like and so on? This is all critically important.

That's because it's at this critical moment that you decide to take a cigarette, set light to it and inhale the fumes. It's at this critical moment that you decide to perform a series of actions, which no one could ever describe as truly involuntary. You may be performing them in response to age-old influences, which you would rather know nothing about (or at least that's been the case in the past). But there is no way that what you are actually doing about any one particular critical moment (and smoking is no more than the result of a series of such moments, interspersed with habit) can be either unconscious or inevitable.

Take your time looking at the personal chart that gets you to this critical moment of choice. Take your time thinking about your personal critical moment. Wallow in your awareness of it. Learn all you can about it. Recognise the ingredients as you would your identical twin. Immerse yourself in it. Think about it. Go over one in subatomic detail. Analyse it forensically. Look at it like a KGB interrogator, from the front, the back, the side. Take its temperature (using a rectal thermometer). Do a pie chart of it. Make a graph of one. DNA-test it. Put it into a centrifuge. Bite it, chew it and spit out the pips.

But whatever else you do, do not overlook it. Your critical moment of choice does what it says on the tin.

Beyond the critical moment

However you choose to illustrate this critical moment on your cartoon chart – and I will leave that entirely to you (though miniature trumpets, highlighters, asterisks and black bordered card all spring to mind) – it should look as though it's forming a point from which two arms or paths will then shoot off. By this, I mean that the overall drift of your progress should be starting to move towards a section that is going to end up looking like the letter 'Y'. Up until now, your life will have been shown following a single path to this point (which point, we shouldn't forget, is reached over and over again, maybe many times a day, but there's no easy way of representing that). Now, by showing two branching routes, you are adding to the picture a recognition of the existence of the alternatives that spring up: a recognition that there will always be two possible ways of moving on from that inevitable 'critical moment'.

I don't suppose that it will come as a huge surprise to you when I say that the two alternative routes are going to take you in quite different directions (hence the Y-shape, which clearly illustrates the ever-widening gap between the first option and the second).

When you reach the critical moment of choice you make a decision which takes you down one route, rather than another. So to make that clear on your chart you now need to draw something which will show the moment of the decision itself and what the decision amounts to, and also what direction the route you're choosing is taking you in.

Route One

Draw your matchstick self on your chart, holding your cigarette in hand. Then, in a way that seems suitably dramatic and significant to you (after all, this is a life-changing event), somehow mark down the fact that, at this critical moment, you are taking the decision to set light to it, and to inhale the fumes. For example, drawing a picture of an old fashioned industrial factory at the side of you, complete with chimney belching out clouds of smoke, would perhaps be an appropriate way to do that.

Once you've drawn yourself putting the decision into action, what about showing the direction that decision is taking you in? How can you do that, and at the same time indicate that this decision you're taking, to smoke the cigarette, is one that you take over and over again, quite probably several times a day? Here are two ideas that should work, but if something else works better for you, go for it. The picture must work for you.

You could try showing your route as:

- A deep-rutted cart track. You've gone down it so many times that the tracks are too deep for you to get out of them. Once you've got stuck in a rut, you're also stuck with the direction that it's taking you in. (You've been smoking for years and years and you don't know how you're going to stop, though you're getting quite desperate about it by now.)

Or:

- A newly surfaced motorway. A route that has been upgraded and upgraded in line with your ever-increasing demand for it, until it has become so smooth and mind-numbingly boring that you sink into a virtually comatose state when you're driving along it. (You hardly notice you're smoking any longer, it's become so automatic and unfulfilling that you need to wake up to what you're doing.)

Whatever image you use it should make it very clear that once you have lit up (every time you have lit up), you have committed yourself to an inevitable direction, one from which you can't alter course.

Next, you need to make sure that as you draw your route on your chart you also make it clear that you know where it's going to end up. Whichever way you've shown it, whether as a well-worn track, a sodium-lit motorway (or something else entirely), draw appropriate road signs (or other signs) to go alongside it. We should all know where we're going when we start off in any particular direction, and if we have been ignoring the signs we shouldn't fool ourselves that we didn't know they existed. After all, ignorance is no defence in the eyes of the traffic police.

The inevitable destination

So where have you been making for every time you've lit up? When you had those early cigarettes, perhaps you didn't think you were going anywhere and believed, like many of us, that you could control the habit? Perhaps you coughed a bit, didn't like the taste and thought you would jack it in, but then 'somehow' didn't? Then, bit by bit perhaps, the habit grew until even you had finally to recognise that you had been going in a direction and that was the direction of becoming that thing you thought you could never be – *a smoker.*

And, once you turned into that smoker, your final destination also became fixed. That's because smokers lose their individuality when they smoke. *All* smokers are going the same way and *all* smokers are going to end up in the same place. The only thing that varies from smoker to smoker, and for any one smoker over the course of their smoking career, is the scale of their destination. For some people (or at an early stage in their smoking career), the destination might be on the scale of a small village, whilst for others (or at a later stage) it might be on the scale of a huge industrial city – we're stuck with the analogy now.

As we're stuck with it, we'll try to make sense of the various end results of smoking behaviour by seeing them as places, which are found at our destination. We'll take them one by one, and as we do you can work out what you have to say about yourself in connection with each one, and then write the results (or an abbreviated version of them) on your 'road sign'. Because you need to recognise that this is where you're making for *every time you light up*.

Pleasure

Where are you going in terms of pleasure as you light up? Well, in the first place, none of us would smoke if we didn't get some pleasure from it, so it's best not to pretend that this part of our destination is going to seem all grim and grey to us. Lighting that cigarette takes us to where we think we want to be, even if it's only for a short time, perhaps as we take our very first drag. It's a place where smokers go to get a little frisson of comfort and calm, somewhere relaxing and liberating. Or it holds out the promise of being that.

But what is the pleasure destination really like, and how long do you stay in it? Because it's usually only available for a short visit. You get there, the sun comes out over that lovely comforting and calming view for a brief moment, then the rain comes down and you have to be on your way. And that means you have to keep repeating the journey in the hope of getting another quick glimpse before the inevitable soaking and driving away.

What do you have to write about your own particular experience of this destination? Has it changed at all over time? Do you really enjoy being there in the way you once thought you did, or are you always hoping to get something out of it that just isn't there? Hasn't any pleasure you once got from smoking become totally lost in the endless search you make to repeat it? Be sure you're being honest about the actual pleasure you get (as opposed to the imagined) when you write about this on your 'road sign'.

Health

Where has your health been going every time you've taken the decision to light up? Before you write anything down for this, you need to remember what your health was like before you started smoking, so you can recognise where you have come from and gone to.

Start with your lungs: you probably had good lungs when you first set out on the route that you choose when you light a cigarette, but what about now? Perhaps the place they first went to when you lit up could have been called Little Tickle in the Throat, a quietish country village sort of a place, but what about now? Is your journey more like a congested struggle towards the Black Country today?

And what about the rest of your body, where is that going? What does your skin look like these days? Is it making visible progress towards freshness, tautness and vitality with every cigarette that you smoke? How does your heart feel? Is it moving fast in the direction of being fitter and stronger each time you light up? And have you looked at the colour of the whites of your eyes recently? Where is your health heading? This is a hard one, but write down on your road sign where you think you will end up, in terms of your physical health, if you carry on in this direction.

Wealth

Where has your wealth been making for, inexorably? Be brave and ask yourself how much you had spent on cigarettes by the end of your first six months of smoking (when you'd finally acknowledged that you were that thing – a smoker). Maybe it was a few hundred pounds, or maybe you counted in farthings and threepenny bits back then, but you probably felt you could wave goodbye to it without too much pain.

However painless it may have felt and whatever the overall state of your finances in those (distant?) days or now, one thing is for sure: the sum total of your wealth has suffered with each decision you've taken to light up. To discover where you've been going financially, just try to add up how much your bank balance has been harmed by your smoking. Has it been by the cost of an exotic foreign holiday a year, or by the cost of a small house? And then think of where you might have got to, if you'd bought a small house in Liverpool with that money a few years ago. Certainly in the good books of your bank manager.

Self-esteem

Where has your chosen route of lighting up at the critical moment taken you in terms of your self-esteem? However you may have felt when you first started lighting up (and, as an addictive type, your self-esteem can never have been of the greatest), by now you must feel as if you've volunteered to take yourself on a route march to Grimly at the Bottom.

For a start, you want to stop smoking (otherwise, presumably, you wouldn't be reading this), and so far haven't been able to. And that in itself is unlikely to improve your self-esteem, as ongoing failure always leaves us feeling inadequate and bad about ourselves. On top of which, you're probably aware of the possibility (probability, in fact) that many non-smokers will be feeling hostile towards you, even if they don't actually say as much. And it doesn't matter what some smokers say about not giving a damn what people think, we're all – smokers and non-smokers alike – only human. We *all* prefer admiration to criticism. Is there anybody whose self-esteem could possibly be improved by the sniping and critical comments that all smokers voluntarily expose themselves to these days? And as smokers are vulnerable in the first place – otherwise they wouldn't be turning to chemical substances to get their needs met – well, it's easy to work out that it's a 'Catch 22' situation.

So write down on your 'road sign' where you think your self-esteem is heading right now. Or, better still, you could draw a picture of yourself standing on a ladder on the sign. Your position on the rungs is where you think you are now and where you're heading can be indicated with an arrow. That's what lighting up means for you.

And that's a very short resumé of where the smoker's chosen route – Route One – takes them each time they reach the critical moment and then light that cigarette. Each time a smoker takes that decision to light up, they choose the deeply rutted path, or the smooth-surfaced motorway that will take them towards the promise of a little, short-lived pleasure, and the certainty of long-term damage to health, wealth and self-esteem.

To keep the analogy going, if we carry on smoking for years, we will inevitably find that the seemingly innocent place we were searching for when we first started smoking has disappeared forever, swamped by the mills and the factories of our increasingly industrialised smoking habit.

We may never be able to return to exactly where or how we were before we started smoking, but we do have the incredibly lucky chance to get back to the all-important critical moment, to the point of choice. Wherever we're at now, whether we're long-time smokers or recently taken to the weed, heavy smokers or occasional ones, we've all still got an equal opportunity to change the route we take at the critical moment, whenever we choose to. And, encouragingly, whatever our current state of health, wealth, or self-esteem, it's still possible for us to improve it. Becoming a smoker usually takes us some time, but it's miraculous just how quickly we can turn ourselves back into being non-smokers again, and then start the process of rebuilding our health, wealth and self-esteem.

And the reason that it can be so quick is that **at any time**, next week, tomorrow, or in the next five minutes, we can choose Route Two, instead of Route One, to take us away from the critical moment. We can then choose to go down Route Two every single time we come to that critical moment, and if we make that choice every single time we hit a critical moment, we become a *non-smoker*. It's as simple as that.

Route Two

If you've ever tried to stop smoking in the past you will already be a little bit familiar with this route. You might feel that you 'sort of' know what the beginning of the journey looks like. You might also 'sort of' know where it should take you to in the end, but of course you won't know what the destination is like for certain, because you haven't been all the way to the end yet. If you had, you would already have stopped smoking.

Maybe what went wrong when you tried it in the past was that you felt the route was not quite your choice; perhaps someone was trying to force you on to it and it didn't feel 'right' for you at the time. If we feel we're being made to try going someone else's way (even if it's obviously a good way), we will usually resist doing it somehow. Often we'll find ourselves saying something like, 'Now's just not the time. I'll know when it comes.'

But this time things are different because this *is* the time. You've chosen to be here, at the starting point to Route Two. So when you look ahead and start to sketch this new route in on the chart, try to forget whatever it was that you saw in its place the last time, otherwise you'll probably end up drawing a route that's difficult, unclear and painful, something that resembles the overgrown, bramble-blocked path in *The Sleeping Beauty*.

This time, you want the route to feel clear, straightforward and as smooth as you're going to be comfortable with. It's *your* way and you want to feel good about sticking to it. So make it look as lovely and rewarding as you want it to be. It's *your* life, and it's *your* future. Live your dream.

Start by deciding what kind of scenery you want around you as you go on this new journey. Is there some special landscape, whether it's a piece of beautiful countryside, an elegant city boulevard, a dramatic coastal path, or some other, either welcoming and cosy or glorious and uplifting setting that you love and feel comfortable in? Somewhere perhaps that you've travelled happily and hopefully in the past? You want the picture on your chart to be as enticing as possible, so make it somewhere special and your own.

Once you've thought carefully about how you want your journey to look, then put on to the place in your chart where Route Two is going to run something that will conjure up the place in your mind. Whenever you look at it, you should feel positive, light-hearted and optimistic. Use a postcard perhaps, or a photo of the place, or a souvenir if you have one, anything – but don't leave the space empty. You want the idea of your new journey to seem as real, identifiable and achievable as you possibly can.

Next, think about where you want this route to take you. You won't be going on a journey completely into the unknown, because some of the destinations you're heading for will be mirror images of places we've already talked about. And that means that this journey should feel both familiar and adventurous for you at the same time, but all the same you will have your own personal ambitions for it, which are separate from the others, and you should be thinking about what they are as well. Where do you want to go? What do you want it to look like? Write it all down on 'road signs', just like before. The only difference this time will be that the destinations are all positive ones.

So let's get going. Should we start by looking at the three most inevitable destinations that we'll arrive at if we take Route Two and choose *not* to light up at the critical moment? They're our old friends: health, wealth and self-esteem, but this time they're going to look like mirror images of the previous destinations.

Health
Check your body over again. Where, physically, is your body at right now? Check your lungs and your breathing, your heart, your skin, your eyes, and all the rest again. We're not promising miracles, but certainties (assuming you have no current malignant disease, but even if you do, then never lighting up again can only be helpful for you). At whatever point your health is now, even if some damage has already taken place, once you've gone down Route Two and stopped lighting those

cigarettes, it will improve. Your lungs *will* grow in capacity, your heart will get stronger and your skin *will* get clearer. When you repeatedly come out of the 'critical moment' on this route, and bypass the lighting-up route, you will find that your body is actually becoming functionally younger. How's that for a promise? – time travel!

Draw a picture on your chart of how you want this new, revitalised, you to be. Take ownership of it. Okay, so it's not easy to draw in the skin of a matchstick person; but you can show yourself jumping about (for the first time since when?); running a marathon (with all that improved lung capacity); singing an aria (with those cleaner vocal chords); playing with your children, or even with the grandchildren that you might now live to see. Use your imagination, but see yourself as doing whatever you want to do, and being, physically, wherever it is you want to be.

Wealth

This is clearly a mirror image of the road already travelled. Have a look back at what you calculated you've lost to cigarettes, and now plan for how you're going to spend all those new savings. Add up the cost of each pack of cigarettes you won't be buying. Think of how lovely those five-pound notes will look all packed together in bundles. How long will it be before you've saved enough to have a trip to the cinema – 24 hours? How long before you can afford a trip abroad – a couple of months? How long before you can afford an investment apartment, a gold ingot, or a retirement plan?

Draw a picture of how you really want to spend all those savings. This is going to be new money, you're going to be making it for yourself, so go on and spend it in ways that will feel good to you. Leave the other money to pay the bills (unless, of course, you were using that for cigarettes ... oh dear). And if it makes the planned excitement more real for you, use the collage technique again. Find bits and pieces, snips of this and that and stick them on to your chart to show what you're going to spend your money on. Use some fabulous material to suggest all the new designer clothes you can have, an advertiser's logo for the sports car you've always just dreamed of, a gourmet food label for all the glorious and exotic foodie treats you can give yourself. Go to town and really, *really* enjoy spending your new-found wealth.

Self-esteem

Perhaps you can draw a ladder for this again, and indicate whereabouts you think you are on the ladder at the moment, and where you want to be. The only difference from the last time you did this will be the direction of the arrow you draw. And, of course, your sense of what is going to be possible, because the further down the ladder you are now, the greater the feeling of achievement will be as you make your way up it. And where else can you possibly go but up when you stop smoking? Stopping smoking is one of the greatest and most achievable feel-good factors you can give yourself. It will almost be worth having started smoking, just so you can have the brilliant feeling that comes with stopping it. No, don't take that literally, it's like saying that getting beaten up is great ... when it stops. But what you can take literally is the fact that at any future 'critical moment', you will be holding your self-esteem in your own hands. And so long as you keep that cigarette in your hands and choose not to put it to your lips, you will be developing your self-esteem, not destroying it.

More than that, just think of the swelling sense of pride when you can look all your old critics in the eye and say, 'I've stopped smoking. Yes, really. For good.'

Don't stint yourself, wallow in that moment. Think of the person (or people) you most want to tell that you've stopped smoking, think of your self-satisfaction, think of the look in their eyes. Then draw a picture of yourself right at the top of that ladder, giving a victory salute.

Pleasure
You didn't think I was going to overlook this, did you?

It won't be all work and no play. You're not going to be dull when you give up smoking, just the opposite. So forget about little breaks in the clouds and add something to your chart that will show you how pleasure can really feel. Give yourself an idea of how much genuine enjoyment you're going to get out of life, now that the guilt, the permanent sense of lack of fulfilment, the unease, the shortness of breath and the carbon monoxide have all gone. Think of all the extra time you're going to have when they're out of the way, and decide how you want to spend it.

Apart from the time you will want to spend contemplating the sheer pleasure of being you, *clever* you, *successful* you, *non-smoker* you, there will be time (and energy) to do so many things when you've stopped smoking. Whatever they are, describe them in all their glorious detail to yourself.

Perhaps you might decide to go running: then, not only will you have the pleasure of actually being able to, without the humiliation of collapsing in a pink, gasping heap, you'll also be able to enjoy the 'high' of the exercise itself; the beauty of the countryside in the early morning or the warm summer evening; the fun of being superior to your friends; most of all, the feel of your own body, working.

Perhaps (now you can afford to) you might decide to spend more time at the cinema, in the theatre, or in galleries or museums. How much more pleasure are you going to get from places like these, when you can concentrate on where you're going and what you're seeing, without all that panicking about wanting to find a place where you can have a cigarette?

Then what about the increased pleasure you're going to get from food and drink? When you can finally taste it properly again, that is. No more dulled taste-buds, no more hollow-mouthed aftertaste, just pure sensation. And you might even find that some curries actually taste hotter than they did!

And then there's the kissing and personal closeness, how have they fitted in with your smoking life up to now? Unless all the people that you've got close to have also been smokers, you will have had problems with intimacy whilst you've been smoking – if only because you will have had the decency to feel that, by smelling bad, you were causing unpleasantness to someone you cared about. Imagine the guilt-free pleasure you can enjoy from now on. You will be able to dive into relationships without all that endless tooth-brushing, gum-chewing and mint-sucking. You will be able to deal with the world without all that self-consciousness.

I'll leave you to think up all the dozens of other ways your pleasure in life and in living is going to increase. It's your destination you're working on, so make sure that you market it well to yourself. You'll love it when you get there.

Your chart is complete now. You've finished putting stick drawings, scraps of fabric and postcards on to it for the time being, and I hope you've had fun. But you may yet want to add a few final flourishes when you finish reading the book. Because the time will have come when you should be able to scatter some gold stars around the end of Route Two. You will have reached your final destination, the golden city, your holy grail. You will be a non-smoker. And you will want to celebrate.

Keep your drawings, pin them up somewhere. They'll be there to remind you of what you've been through, what it takes to be successful, and of what success finally looks like.

Your choice

You've just finished examining the two alternative routes that you can take whenever you reach a 'critical moment of choice'. With all the work you've been doing on your chart you should be able to see, very graphically and clearly, where your better option lies. And it would be pretty odd if you couldn't see what most people see, which is that the choice is a no-brainer. In fact, right now you may be absolutely convinced that you've totally seen the light and that you've stopped smoking forever – which would be absolutely brilliant. But even if you are convinced there is still work to be done, and if you haven't quite reached that state of belief yet, there are definitely more things that need to be thought about. It's onwards and upwards all the way from here, though. You've progressed most of the way towards achieving all the skills you're going to need to stop smoking, and all we're going to be working on now is staying stopped.

Practice makes perfect

Mozart may have been a genius musician and John McEnroe may have had a natural talent for tennis, but neither of them got where they are today without practice, practice, practice. We all just get surprisingly better and better at doing something when we do it over and over again. The same goes for doing the wrong thing as well. Which means that a smoker, someone who has always got to the critical moment and taken Route One, where they light up and end up sicker, poorer and sadder, has become very well-practised in doing just that. They've become a world expert at it, got used to the whole idea, and generally become totally professional at what they're doing. To become non-smokers, first we all have to 'unpractise' smoking, and then we have to practise doing the other thing, that is to say making the choice of Route Two, which will take us in the direction of health, wealth and happiness, at the critical moment. We have to actively learn how to do the thing we really want to do all along. It sounds absurd, doesn't it? But that's how our minds work.

Now I'm not suggesting that you stand for hours looking at a packet of cigarettes, willing yourself not to have one. Nor am I suggesting that you keep taking a few out and tempting yourself by popping them in and out of your mouth. You've probably got better things to do with your time. But what I am suggesting you do is reprogramme yourself internally.

To do this you need to take yourself to the edge, that is, the 'critical moment', in a variety of 'worst case scenarios'. You know, those times when you had to have a cigarette in the past, and (if you're being ruthlessly honest with yourself) you suspect you might still be gasping for one in the future. Then, having mentally immersed yourself in all that the moment has to offer – all the stress, all the emotional and chemical overload, and all the pre-programmed habitual behaviour of grabbing for that packet of fags – you can start to 'flick' between the two alternative routes out of it, keeping the final destinations of both firmly in mind as you do it.

It's very important that this process is worked through. When we stop smoking, we get over the nicotine craving really very quickly, but we don't stop having ghostly visitations of the craving for the habit, and – this is the really significant bit – we don't stop feeling the same old need to have our emotions cared for and soothed. Cigarettes have for a long time been our preferred way to handle that, so, as well as stopping smoking, we need to desensitise ourselves to the link between cigarettes and emotional neediness. If we don't do that, we put ourselves at risk of relapse whenever we get back into a situation where we've been used to soothing ourselves with a ciggie.

So that's our immediate job now, to desensitise ourselves. Very soon, after that, we'll go on to explore the various other ways we might start to get those needs met (two books for the price of one!).

Target Practice
Or, A short and practical guide to desensitising

This business of desensitising has a chapter all to itself simply because it needs to stand out. It won't take long to read – it's the shortest chapter in this book – but it might take rather longer to do.

The first thing you need to do in the desensitisation process is to think back to all the information you've gathered about yourself and your smoking history, and decide on a situation that would typically have had you gasping for a ciggie. If you think of yourself as a social smoker, for example, that situation could be when you find yourself in the pub with your mates, after work, on a Friday night. If you've decided you're a 'trauma' smoker, on the other hand, a typical situation would come at a time of crisis; if you're a rebel smoker, it would come when you're angry – hopefully you get the picture of what's needed.

Having decided on a typical situation, here's what to do next.

1 Make sure you're on your own and unlikely to be disturbed.

2 Make sure that there are no cigarettes available.

3 Make yourself comfortable, have a pleasant drink to hand (but avoid alcohol, it messes with your commitment).

4 Target a memory of some particular time when you felt yourself getting really stressed-out because you were in a 'typical' situation, with your trigger feelings were all in place. Your trigger moment had come and you had to face the critical moment of choice. Of course, at that particular time you did actually have a cigarette. But this time you're going to practise staying with the moment, immersing yourself in it, flicking back and forth between the two alternative routes, and then coming out of the moment again, having taken Route Two and rejected the cigarette.

Remember the visualising technique we used earlier in the book? As you do all this, run it through in your mind as if it was a video. So that you end up both 'in yourself', and able to feel your feelings, and at the same time, 'out of yourself' and able to see the action as if it was on film.

5   Keep rewinding the video and replaying the moment. Play with your feelings, try on the old ones again and again, and then allow yourself the sensation of being aware that you're letting yourself down, again and again. Then try the alternative route, feel the feeling, and don't do it anyway. Allow yourself to hold yourself in the moment without giving in to the 'overwhelming' feeling. Start to build up a familiarity with what it will feel like to have overcome the hurdle successfully. Start to become familiar with the extraordinarily powerful relief of success.

6   Breathe deeply and steadily.

7   And allow yourself a smile.

8   Practise doing this over and over again at other times until you can feel fairly sure that you have desensitised yourself to the needy feelings in that particular situation, and have familiarised yourself with an alternative way of dealing with the situation.

9   When you're feeling really strong and ready, and not before, put yourself into a situation that is as close to the original as you can, but take a willing and confidential friend with you for support (but not to 'control' you or 'make' you do the right thing). Then go through the process consciously and describe what you're doing and feeling to your friend as you're going through it.

10 Buy your friend a drink and have one for yourself.

Congratulations, you have now immersed yourself in a situation that previously would have ended with you smoking, and you've come out without lighting up. I think we can safely say you are now a non-smoker.

Smoking Replacement Therapy
Or, It'll be a positive pleasure

The rest of the book is really all about support systems and alternative ways of getting your emotional needs met, so that you're less likely to be looking for that chemical crutch in the first place.

We hear that nature abhors a vacuum, and to a large extent we have actually been creating a vacuum by what we've been doing with this book. We have been looking at the ingredients of smoking and trying to remove them, one by one, which, of course, will mean that where each one was before we'll be left with an empty space. And if we're left with a space that nature wants us to fill, it will be only too easy for us to fill it with something as undesirable as smoking has been in the past. Think how many people just end up gorging themselves on chocolate, crisps and burgers when they've quit smoking, which then leave them feeling unwell and make them put on so much weight that they finally rush to pick up the ciggies again.

So, rather than just leaving you with the empty spaces where smoking used to be, and abandoning you to sink or swim when you're faced with them, we're going to look at ways of filling those spaces with something more useful and desirable than smoking ever was. We're going in for some smoking replacement therapy.

Please note: this should not be confused with nicotine replacement therapy. Nicotine replacement therapy works to help us overcome our short-term dependence on the chemical 'feel-good' factor in a cigarette, but it does nothing to help us overcome our dependence on all the other ingredients of smoking behaviour. Nor does it do anything to help us overcome our dependence on the cigarette itself, with all the significance that has for us as part of our daily ritual and all the associations it might have with, say, good times with friends, or glamour, or being slim.

Nor does nicotine replacement therapy have anything substantial to offer in terms of helping us to deal with those strong emotional needs we have, the ones that have always been covered up behind the smokescreen of a cigarette in the past.

What we are offering here is *smoking* replacement therapy, which is quite a different matter. Smoking replacement therapy does what it says. It provides a replacement for all the aspects and ingredients of smoking behaviour. Nicotine replacement therapy might, for some people, make up part of the package, but it can never be more than that – a part of the overall package.

If smoking replacement therapy is to succeed in providing a replacement for all the ingredients of smoking behaviour, we must, first of all, look back and remind ourselves of just what that smoking behaviour has been doing for us and what it has been providing us with all this time. Once we're certain of all that, then – and only then – can we also be certain that any new alternatives we come up with will be what we need, and will not simply leave us with another space, another problem to sort out later.

Cigarettes and smoking provide us, most obviously, with chemicals that temporarily soothe our emotions and our mood. This is the part of smoking behaviour that nicotine replacement therapy can, sometimes, help us with. In addition, as we've seen a thousand times, cigarettes and smoking give us 'something to do' with ourselves. We'll get on to those areas, and to the alternatives that can be found for them, in a little while. But before we get on to the physical aspects of smoking behaviour, we're first going to look back at the underlying emotional needs that have been demanding all along that we do something about them. The ones that smoking has been doing such a great cover-up job for.

Managing those needy feelings

You'll remember that on page 32 I explained that the basic response mechanisms to stimulation and stress are poorly adapted in addictive people. (Go back and re-read it, to remind yourself, if you need to.) I also said that such people were addicted to their own behaviour, but that there were ways that this could be managed and that I would explain later the ways in which this could be done.

Well, we've arrived at 'later', and so now we're going to be looking for ways to manage those uncomfortable feelings, the ones that make us squirm. And note the language: I'm saying 'manage', meaning 'cope with' them, without trying to cover up for them by reaching for a pack of cigarettes. We're not attempting to achieve something as revolutionary as killing off the feelings. It isn't realistic to imagine that we are actually going to completely reinvent ourselves and our body's responses, so that we become capable of responding to situations with floods of different chemicals. Well, certainly not immediately – and probably not without intensive psychological re-education. But it is realistic to think that we can learn immediately to 'swallow' the agitating hormones (not literally, of course), using techniques such as deep breathing and basic relaxation. By this means, we can give ourselves time to come up with different, and more controlled, emotional and physical behaviours than we have done in the past.

If it helps, try to think of the process this way: imagine you're like a hungry small boy who is in a supermarket. The child has to learn to cope with both his hunger and his sense of frustration when he is prevented from grabbing food and eating it straight from the shelves. The first time it happens, the child can't manage his feelings and so yells blue murder. On subsequent visits, he is still likely to feel hungry but, with time, he learns to live with his feelings, control his behaviour and wait until his hunger can be satisfied in a more acceptable way. And one of the greatest things that a carer can do for a child under those circumstances is to turn the child's attention on to something else, whilst his emotions have the chance to be brought under control again.

People who have stopped smoking have to learn to do the same thing, that is, to bring their emotions under control again. There's no point in our pretending that the old sensations are just going to end up in the bin along with the cigarette packets. We are still as likely as ever to experience all the same agitating chemicals in all the same old stress situations. But the sensations that the chemicals create can be lived with – after all, they're not going to kill us, are they? And, like any small child, with enough other distractions to keep our minds off them we'll get past the point when they're overwhelming us. And we can get there without having to smoke.

Now, I can just hear someone saying, 'I'm not some kind of raging animal. I liked having a smoke, that's all. How come you're telling me I'm supposed to hold in all these non-existent floods of emotion before I can give up for good.'

To which I can only say, 'If there's nothing big going on behind it all, why hasn't it been easy for you to give up?'

The thing is that we've all become so used to having these strong emotional needs that they've come to seem normal to us, even when they've really been at the extreme end of the average spectrum of sensations. I mean, some people actually think it's normal to poke short white sticks, which are full of dried-up leaves, into their mouths, set them on fire, and then breathe in their toxic smoke, all so they can feel relaxed enough to 'have a good time'! What does that say about the emotional state they're in when they're in company?

So, it's back to the emotional drawing board.

Near the beginning of this book, on page 20, I asked some questions, which should have got you thinking about what, emotionally speaking, you really want from life. They came under the heading, 'What do you get out of smoking?', and they made suggestions of various feelings that you might have believed you were satisfying whenever you smoked a cigarette. Or, to put it another way, they offered you 'reasons' for smoking. Go back and look at those questions, and also look back at the answers you gave, detailing which feelings were being satisfied when you smoked. Then look at your replies. You will probably find that these are telling you what your emotional neediness has really been demanding all along. Your emotional neediness has almost certainly actually been a need to fix this, or these, particular feelings (the ones you've detailed), rather than a need to smoke a cigarette after all.

Alternative pleasures

To make my meaning clearer and also to be more specific, let's use the example of, 'I feel this is one of my few pleasures in life' as one of the main emotional rewards you could have felt you got from smoking cigarettes. Now ask yourself if the basic, underlying problem with this one isn't so much that you lack pleasures in your life (you feel you have only a few), but that your *desire* for pleasures is not being dealt with. Let's face it, lots of nuns and monks will have gone for years and years without many obvious pleasures in their lives, and some of them will have been happy enough bunnies all the same. Why not you? Because you have a stronger desire for pleasure, that's all (and there's nothing wrong in that).

And if the problem is that the desire for pleasure is not being dealt with, then why not satisfy it? If we're looking for pleasure, what we're really looking for is more sensory stimulation, which is a way of saying we're looking to get physical feedback that will give us 'emotional strokes'. In other (and much simpler) words, pleasure is a way of making ourselves 'feel good'. And when we think of all the possible ways in the world that we might get sensory stimulation, emotional strokes and more of the feel-good factor into our lives, isn't cigarette smoking pretty close to the bottom of a list of good ways to deal with it?

So what we really need if we've written, 'I feel this is one of my few pleasures in life,' is to spend *more* time getting *more* sensory stimulation. And while we're at it, let's let our imaginations run riot and come up with some rather more exciting ideas than having a fag.

Meeting physical needs

If you want more pleasure in life, how about:

- Having your skin soothed and stroked with exotic, relaxing, perfumed oils, whilst having a glorious full body massage (at a cost of no more than four packets of cigarettes, or infinitely less at your local college).

- Lying in a steaming, herb-fragranced bath, in a room that glows with the light of dozens and dozens of tea lights or candles, whilst listening to gentle jazz.

- Having a sauna or steam bath, followed by a plunge into an energising icy tub (it makes your brain work better as well as your body, and will cost less than the price of two packets of fags).

- Preparing and eating, all by yourself, a most carefully planned and beautifully presented organic meal, which mixes delicate flavours with intriguing textures.

- Running barefoot on a sharply sandy beach, or over springy, short-cropped, heath or downland (this one's free).

- Sharing exquisitely tactile time with someone special, tracing patterns on each other's bodies with feathers or with paintbrushes (spend longer and paint a picture, why not?).

Find as many of your own ways to get more sensory pleasure into your life as there are days in the week and weeks in the year. The main thing is to feel that you're *entitled* to have this kind of pleasure and then the ideas will flow. And the great beauty of it all is that when you do allow yourself to enjoy more genuine sensory pleasure you will no longer feel a need for things like cigarettes, which only serve to block your full sensory enjoyment.

Those ideas could work just as well to fulfil various other emotional needs besides the need for pleasure, but they're not catch-alls, and it just isn't technically possible to list every emotionally fulfilling alternative to cigarettes that might exist. Apart from anything else, to work for each one of us, ideas should really come from us as individuals, but as there are times when we all need a little help with inspiration, there follow one or two suggestions for each of the other categories on the list.

Meeting emotional needs

Only a robot doesn't need emotional fulfilment of any kind, but some of our needs are complex, and less healthy than is good for us. What has your particular brand of emotional neediness been demanding that you have tried to cover up with cigarettes? Back to the list on page 20.

I feel calmer

What you're really saying here is that you're overloaded and find it hard to cope, which is why you get worked up. What you actually need to do about this is to learn to accept things more, and that should especially include learning to accept yourself and your limitations more. A cigarette won't help you to accept yourself, just the opposite. Why not try yoga instead, with a little meditation thrown in?

I feel life is more bearable

Why is it so unbearable at the moment? Perhaps you need to look at things a bit differently, and get a new (and more philosophical) perspective on life? Try re-framing and rethinking the way you see the world with an NLP (neuro-linguistic programming) course, or cognitive behavioural counselling. Or travel to somewhere there is real deprivation to discover just how much people can actually cope with when they have to.

I feel less lonely; that I've got a friend

If you're feeling lonely, that could be because, even though there are people around, you feel you're nothing unless you're in a very close relationship, that you need someone else to 'complete you'. Or it could be simply because there is no one around. But cigarettes aren't company. Try a dog, a cat, a parrot instead or, better still, enrol in some classes and become more interesting to yourself (you'll find you'll become more interesting to others then, as well). Join a dating or general introduction agency, non-smokers are more sought after.

I feel I'm being defiant – and to hell with it

I think we've already covered this. If you always need to challenge and take on authority, try to become an authority yourself. It's the only way you'll be happy. Teach somebody something that you know a lot about. You'll find it a better way to even things up than killing yourself with a cigarette. And by passing on knowledge that is appreciated, you get that sense of being validated and really counting for something that you've been looking for all along.

I feel I'm allowed to be angry

There's a lot of this about. We're usually angry when we think something in life is unfair. Learn to question why you feel everything has to be fair in the first place. Work on developing a philosophy that includes a greater acceptance of the varying standards, attitudes and behaviours in life that we all have to deal with. Spend more time around animals: they won't ask for fairness, just for strokes.

I feel sexy

Well, we would probably all like to feel sexy, but what this is saying is that you don't really feel sexy in your own skin, you think you need props. It wasn't a cigarette that made Marlene Dietrich sexy, it was all the rest of the package that was her. So why not work on developing the other things that go with 'sexy'? The voice, the body language, the grooming. And if you're a woman who needs props, how about a satin and lace basque? That would only be a killer in one respect. Or, if you're a chap, how about developing a solid six-pack? So much sexier than a 20-pack.

I feel grown up

If you think cigarettes make you grown up, that means you feel very young in the first place. And what's wrong with feeling young? Well, everything, when you're young, and nothing when you're older! Smoking isn't grown up, it's kids who smoke most, so the more you smoke, the younger you look. Grown-up people are giving up in ever greater numbers. If you really want to feel grown up, you could always try taking out a mortgage and a pension, and the dog before work.

I feel macho

See above, re developing a solid six-pack. Dying of cancer doesn't make anyone feel, or look, macho. If you're copying the behaviour of someone you think of as being macho, ask yourself if there isn't something else they do that is genuinely more macho than puffing desperately on a fag. Try out the parts of their behaviour that you genuinely find admirable, avoid the rest, and don't be afraid to be your own man. Macho is as macho does. Be brave enough to reject things that aren't good for you.

I feel less anxious

Here I have to admit that cigarettes *do* help to relieve anxiety, but only for about 30 seconds, after which they'll leave you feeling more anxious. But what you're really saying (just as in 'I feel calmer') is not that you're looking to treat anxiety, but that you're looking for solutions to it. You need to learn how not to be anxious in the first place. Smokers are anxious people, so don't hang around them, they'll only make anxiety seem normal. Watch non-anxious people, you'll find that one of their secrets is that they take more notice of the outside world, and obsess and talk less about themselves than anxious people do. Try yoga and anything that will focus your mind. Become more interested in what people think, and less in what they think about you.

I feel soothed

So why were you so agitated? Couldn't you try being soothed by spending time in someone else's company? Or try to develop relationships with more soothing people, or try any of the ideas listed under 'I feel this is one of my few pleasures in life'. Go for long walks in the country, or start reading poetry aloud to yourself (especially rhythmic and rhymed poetry). You don't have to 'go slow' in life, just learn to pace yourself more, and be prepared to consider a less 'exciting' (often another way of saying frightening, confrontational or over stimulating) lifestyle.

I feel I've got time out

Does that mean actively having time for yourself? Or, more negatively, having time when you can make all of the rest of the world, together with its demands, go away? Either way, the root of the problem may be that you don't feel in control of your world, you feel dominated and tyrannised by it. Which, in turn, could mean that you have unrealistic expectations of how much control it is possible for anyone to have. Or it could mean that your way of looking at things is skewed towards concentrating on what you can't control, rather than towards what you can control. Smoking a cigarette won't make time, it's just another way of making yourself a slave. Try growing plants (even a window box can produce herbs), as a way to get time out of the rat race. Growing vegetables lets you take charge of your own means of production, and it's a lesson in taking things at nature's pace, for better or worse.

I feel I belong

To what? – part of the pack? Maybe that pun says enough about the absurdity, and pathos, of feeling that you can belong because of a *cigarette*. Of course, what you're really after is a sense that you matter somehow. And rather than mattering because you can offer something of genuine value to the world, you choose to matter by going in for 'pack behaviour' (sorry, that old pun again). You're not a dog (or a cigarette), so why not aim to become more interesting and valuable in your own right? Provide people with something they can genuinely value and enjoy, something they will come asking for. Play the piano, learn massage, read palms, make really good foodie treats, become an expert in tax returns, learn how to tell a joke well – these are all ways of becoming hugely attractive and valuable to others.

I feel less fat

This is top of so many wish lists! But smoking doesn't make or keep anyone thin, only eating less and exercising more can do that. Are you sure you haven't bought into the Kate Moss myth, that if you smoke like her, you'll look like her? We won't go into the 'fat' question here; for one thing, that belongs to a separate book, for another it's irrelevant to smoking. Replace the two ingredients that smoking might arguably give you – (1) something to do with your hands and (2) something to take your mind off food – with (1) worry beads or knitting and (2) outdoor exercise, and the job is done. No more excuses.

I feel can concentrate

This is another tricky one, because nicotine does actually have a slightly positive effect on concentration. It does seem to help some chemically unbalanced brains focus better. But why is concentration a problem for you in the first place? Concentration is usually a problem for one of two reasons: either there is something wrong with our brain chemistry, or we feel detached, for some reason, from whatever it is we're working on.

If it's the first, you might be unwell, so get yourself checked out by a doctor. You might also try changing your diet – go for more natural and organic foods, plus plenty of fish oils – and getting more oxygen into your system, through exercise.

If you're not relating to whatever you're working on, is it because you are out of your depth? Or are you bored, or feeling alienated? Work out what the problem may be and talk about it to someone who can help. Work on the underlying problem. Don't just cover it up or create another one for yourself, by resorting to cigarettes.

I feel that it is one of my few pleasures in life
We've done that one – see above.

I feel – I'm enjoying my fag
Maybe you do actually enjoy the taste. I suppose somebody has to. Or perhaps you resent interference and this feeling is a blocking manoeuvre. You may always resist any suggestion that you're not actually enjoying smoking, so I'll restrict myself to saying we can't always have everything that we want. And if you didn't also want something besides cigarettes you wouldn't be reading this now.

Either you genuinely like bitter tastes, in which case learn to love something that tastes as bitter as cigarettes, but is less harmful, like gentian root (it'll purify you at the same time). Or you maybe just like to paddle your own canoe. If you like to do your own thing, then recognise that you've made stopping smoking your own decision and think, 'Well done'. Then stick as bloody-mindedly to enjoying not smoking as you once did to enjoying smoking.

I feel – well, it's just a smoke, isn't it?
There's a sort of fatalism in that, isn't there? Or is it a need to minimise the significance of things in your life? Do you feel that anything you do can't be *that* important? Or is it that you often feel defensive about what you do? In either case, it sounds like there might be an underlying lack of self-confidence. And smoking cigarettes won't do anything to improve that – quite the opposite, in fact.

You need to work on building up a sense that what you do actually *does* matter. That you have the right to value yourself and your achievements more. Start by telling yourself that it's not just a smoke, that it's really a sure way to harm yourself, and that you're worth more than that. That you matter enough to want to take care of yourself. Buy yourself some token thing that you've always wanted but could never see a reason to buy (perhaps a small piece of jewellery, or an expensive ornament) – it'll make a lot more sense than buying a packet of fags!

This next item wasn't on the original list.

It helps at times when I feel my life isn't my own
Actually, that's not what you're likely to be aware of feeling. But something along those lines is likely to underpin a lot of the feelings that smokers have. When we get right back to the foundations of what we're doing, we often find that, in some way, we are responding to other people with our smoking behaviour. Either we want to look 'big' for them, or we're cheesed off with them, or we're copying them, or we're sad because we can't get enough of their company – or, or, or, or … It all boils down to us basing our behaviour on wanting to please or appease others.

Whose life is it anyway? We should make the most of our own lives – and we should each start by doing what's good for *us*.

This section was all about managing emotional needs. Just remember that when you take away the grubby comfort blanket of cigarette smoking you mustn't leave a vacuum. You need to replace it with something more wholesome and generally satisfying that can fit into your life, otherwise you'll only long to fill the empty space with some other form of addiction.

Managing our physical/behavioural needs

Stopping smoking can be one of the hardest things we ever do in life. Smoking cigarettes can be one of the hardest habits to break (even harder than alcohol and drug addiction), and that's not only because nicotine is such a ferocious little chemical, but also because smoking cigarettes provides us with so very many satisfying associations, which we know we're going to have to lose.

We've just been looking at the emotional associations of smoking. We're actually not interested in replacing the chemical ones (except in extreme cases of addiction, in which case nicotine replacement therapy may be of use) because we don't want or need those chemicals anyway. And now the time has come to look at the physical things that cigarette smoking has been bringing into your life. And also to think about what alternative things you can do or get involved in, which will help you to get over missing cigarettes and, at the same time, bring you infinitely more interesting and satisfying ways of spending your time and energy. And now, finally, we're going to consider the lifestyle and ritual associations of smoking.

A lot of people actually find that it helps to stop smoking when they're away on holiday or when they're working to a different schedule from normal. This is because our brains get used to doing things at set times, in set ways, or in set places. We set up associations of mood, setting and behaviour, which become fixed as, 'This is what I do with myself at this time of day and when I feel like this,' ideas in our minds. For example, 'It's 11 o' clock, mmmm, I'm all thought out, I need a coffee and a fag.'

It is because some behaviours, like smoking, can become so 'scheduled' into our lives that when we want to break out of them it will be easier to do it during an overall break in routine. If the lifestyle and ritual associations are already challenged or overturned, it makes it harder for us to stick to the behaviour 'unconsciously'.

It also follows that if we break out of the daily timetable, we give ourselves the chance of avoiding the people we usually get into cahoots with at the back of the office or down at the pub. We can more easily get away from the places and situations that are most likely to 'trip' the sensory associations that smoking will have for us. You're not avoiding anyone for judgmental or moral reasons, just because of the associations they have for you with smoking. We need a chance to desensitise all our old sensory connections so that we can be free to make new ones. You can tell your friends that you still want to spend time with them, but just away from cigarettes, at least for a while. If they're good friends, they'll go along with it (and, actually, probably join you).

Now, let's have a look at what physical 'pleasures' we've been getting from smoking, and see whether or not it's going to be possible to replace any of them, or whether we have to learn simply to go without.

Although we've tripped over them here and there throughout the book, the place we spent longest looking at the rituals and habits that go with smoking cigarettes was the chapter 'It's a Fag'. Now we're going to look again at some of those rituals, bring in some new ones, and find out what they've all been doing for us, in terms of the physical and behavioural rewards that we've got from smoking cigarettes.

Once we've got to grips with those things, we can move on to search out newer, fresher, healthier, and altogether more interesting alternatives to the habit we've had of spending time and money setting fire to gift-wrapped poisons in our mouths.

The ritual pleasures of smoking

We all understand – or we should by now – that a great deal of the 'pleasure' we derive from smoking is bound up in the rituals that surround our habit. The list of these rituals is long and varied.

Buying cigarettes

You have probably had a cigarette-buying habit, even if it's been so loose that you'd only ever describe it as random. Smoking behaviour can sometimes be made to continue for longer than necessary by the simple presence of 'automatically' bought cigarettes in the house; and then, once you've stopped smoking, temptation can be stirred up if you ever go back into cigarette-buying mode. It's easy for us to go into default mode when we're not actively controlling our behaviour, and that can mean that we'll find ourselves walking into whatever paper shop or cigarette kiosk we've been used to buying fags from. Which is particularly irritating and depressing when we've just stopped smoking. But this is one of the many areas that can be positively affected by a break in routine in the early days of stopping smoking. At least if we spend a few days away from home, or just out of our usual routine, we'll be thinking much more consciously about what we're doing all the time, and at the same time avoiding the familiar associations that our usual shop or supermarket is going to stir up.

Another very good tip is to avoid going back to our same old shop, at the same old time, to buy cigarette substitutes, such as chocolates or gum. For one thing, simply dreaming up substitutes and buying them instead of cigarettes doesn't make a break with the addictive ritual itself. For another, chewing sweet and synthetic foodstuffs in place of cigarettes only replaces one addictive and unhealthy substance with another.

If you must have treats, it's best if you make them healthy ones, such as nuts or fruit (which you're likely to buy somewhere slightly different anyway). But if you insist on having syrupy ones (and we might as well be realistic about this), then at least buy them in a different way from the way you used to buy cigarettes. If you bought cigarettes in a sweet shop, buy your treats at the supermarket, and vice versa. But most of all, avoid making impulse purchases of the sweets or other things you're using as substitutes for cigarettes. There are two reasons for this: firstly, as an addictive type you need to practise controlling your 'need' for immediate gratification; and, secondly, by planning your treats you will get more satisfaction and pleasure in the long run. (Plus you will usually be able to source them at a better price and so save money.)

Smoking in time and space

This Einstein-like subheading only refers to the times and places that your behaviour has become ritualised and to the fact that, in certain circumstances, your smoking has ended up associated more with the time of day and the place you're in than with anything else. For example, you might have ritualised your practice of going out of the office, down the back stairs and into the smoking 'bike shed'; or you might have ritualised a 'happy hour' after work, when you were always to be found with a wine glass in one hand and a cigarette in the other. The only significant things involved in what you were doing were the times and places you were doing it.

It's the same story as before: when you want to stick to stopping smoking, you need to break any association there has been between smoking and circumstances. And again, it will help to begin the process by making a change in your day-to-day routine for a time. So, either go away for a few days, or at the very least change enough parts of your routine that you are forced to concentrate that bit harder on what you actually are doing. Concentration is vital to changing rituals. If your usual order of events, when smoking at work, was to go to the loo, then downstairs for a cigarette, don't just remove the cigarette, change the whole order of events of your break times. Make yourself a coffee, drink it, have a natter, but whatever you do, don't go to the loo until near the end of your break. You'll feel you're doing something altogether different, not just going without that cigarette.

And if you still insist on joining your mates for the happy hour (not the very greatest of ideas), at least protect yourself as much as possible from all the old associations with cigarettes. Sit somewhere totally different. Choose drinks with lots of fruit, ice, soda, tonic, or other mixers in them. Make use of the materials in your drink – chew on the ice, or nibble the lemon and, to make your drink last longer, try sipping it through a straw (maybe not such a good idea if you're a guy, however). Don't substitute the cigarette part of the ritual with crisps (the fats and salts in them are addictive, and fattening as well – they'll only make things worse for you). Don't get plastered, otherwise you'll lose the self-awareness and self-control you need to change your rituals. But whatever else you do, break up as much of your previous ritual as you can, and, as soon as possible, replace the lost parts with healthier ones.

Above all, as you make spaces in your routines, remember the following:

- Avoid creating vacuums.

- Fill the spaces with exciting changes and not with poor substitutions.

- Never allow yourself to feel that you're just going to end up with something second best.

- Ritualise new and useful habits so you can feel you're getting something fresh out of this process of stopping smoking.

Ritual as a manual event

This is just a posh way of saying that when you open a pack of cigarettes, take one out, play around with your lighter, light your cigarette, flick your ash into a special container (or on to the floor), stub your ciggie out, chuck the evidence out of the window, and everything else you do when you 'smoke', you're carrying out a series of hand-related activities that amount to an 'event'.

Finding something different to do with our hands is very important, probably vitally so, once we've stopped smoking. But that doesn't mean we should replace the cigarette that was once the darling of our hands with a cigarette substitute to fiddle with, such as a pen. That would be the equivalent of replacing a person with a picture of them – we will only miss the original more. You should aim to keep your hands working in some way – playing with worry beads, fiddling with things (but try not to drive your friends and co-workers mad), squeezing squashy balls, playing with executive toys, working out Rubik's cube, anything that is more than just 'ghost smoking'.

In modern society we don't seem to have nearly as many things to do with our hands as people used to have; there used to be sewing, knitting, polishing things, writing longhand, whittling sticks, making models, building transistor radios – all of these seem to have disappeared and nothing, with the possible exception of texting, that is modern, manual and manipulative has taken their place. We want manual ritual back in our lives.

If you don't find texting that exciting, try to make other things fill the manual gap left by cigarettes. Make life a little bit more (rather than less) manually complicated. For example, change from making instant coffee to creating the full coffee monty; grind your beans, then measure the ground coffee into a jug, carefully add the water, froth the milk while you're waiting, etc., etc. Learn to enjoy using your hands to carry out the full ceremonial and take pride in doing it really well. You can make ceremonies out of tea making, too, like the Japanese do, or as in the full English, complete with tea leaves, bone china, sandwiches and warming the teapot. Alternatively, use your hands for intricate work, like mending watches, or fine construction, such as building card houses. But give your hands a real reason to live other than bashing at a keyboard all day, and they'll have less reason to remember all that fiddling about with fags.

A good tip whilst you're thinking about stopping smoking is to change the hand you usually hold your cigarette with. As a large part of the 'pleasure' of smoking is got from the ritual or habit involved, the more we change of the ritual or habit, the less straightforwardly pleasurable we will find the changed activity. And the easier it will be to break the whole of the habit.

Best of all keep your hands busy in someone else's, or even holding someone else – just till you're past the early stage of missing holding a cigarette, that is!

Oral gratification

From a very early age, we enjoy putting things in our mouths. Anything from stones, to dirt, to our own fingers – or other people's – go into our mouths when we're young, so it's not surprising that eventually some needy people will decide to comfort themselves by sucking on finger substitutes. When you've stopped smoking you will want to start fulfilling old needs in new ways and, sadly, bunging a cigarette-shaped thing into your mouth as a substitute for a cigarette is not going to achieve that. It's only going to keep reminding you of cigarettes themselves. It's better to avoid substitutes entirely and to keep your mouth busy and active in other ways, at least until the 'imprint' of having a cigarette in there has gone.

Your family and friends will probably think you've lost it completely, but a very good way to keep your mouth busy is to keep speaking your thoughts to yourself in an ongoing silent conversation with yourself. Keep mouthing your thoughts silently this way and your mouth will have so much to do it'll forget all about cigarettes.

I'm afraid that gum and mints have become so closely associated with stopping smoking that, unless you've been brought up on Uranus, using them to keep your mouth busy is only likely to keep reminding you of the cigarettes they're replacing (and they're nutritionally challenged and quite addictive anyway). If you do genuinely find that chewing or sucking something helps you get over smoking, then find something different to put in your mouth. Eat chewy fruit and nuts or suck on bits of fruit peel and the teats of water bottles. But overall you'll probably be better off in the long term if you retrain your mouth to live without all that constant non-nutritious stimulation.

Masonic intimacies

When smoking was considered more socially acceptable than it is now, people who smoked could feel that they were connecting themselves to a big social group when they lit up. Now that it is less socially acceptable people who smoke are much more likely to feel they are connecting themselves to a rather furtive, semi-secret society. Or to a group of people who are as much interested in standing up for their individual rights as anything else. Either way, the connection between the people in the group is going to be more about behaviour than about achievement. If what you want is to belong to a rather separatist, or in some way exclusive, group, who go in for a behaviour that brings them together, then when you stop smoking you could try to find another similar group that can meet your needs. But why not make the achievement of something a target instead? Otherwise you might just end up in a nose-pickers society.

Try sharing group activities that bring results – like bands, choirs or theatre groups, which nearly all give performances of some kind. Or if it's the gossipy, 'select' intimacy of the smoking circle that you've enjoyed in the past, try a writing group or a political organisation to get a similar, but more productive, effect. Of course, the probability is that in any of these groups you'll still find smokers, but that shouldn't be more of a problem to you than meeting them in the street. The main point is that if we want to belong to a group (and groups do bring something of real value into our lives), then it's better to join one that has some group target besides the rather sad and unhealthy one (psychologically as well as physically) of smoking cigarettes. We will have the advantages of being in a group but get rid of the disadvantage of having to smoke cigarettes in order to be a member.

The big problem with all those physical and behavioural 'rewards' that smoking has been bringing into our lives, is that each one of them has been both an excuse and a counterfeit. If we had genuine needs, we could have found better ways of fixing them than by smoking poisonous leaves. Cigarettes are the greatest con artists and smoking is the greatest con trick in that world of cigarettes we've shared. Or they would be, except that, as I said before, 'they' have never existed. We have invented them.

By taking time out when we stop smoking, we give ourselves the best chance of un-inventing all the emotional and physical meaning we have associated with the smoking of cigarettes, simply by making the necessary time and space available to break the links.

Don't forget

Notice that I haven't said, at any stage, that we need to take our minds off smoking. A lot of people say that when they're quitting they need to take up something else which will help them forget about their burning desire for cigarettes. The trouble is that when they're saying it they usually put it like this, 'Whenever I stop smoking I find it easier if …', which rather gives the game away – they've never succeeded.

If you mean to give up – for good – you don't actually want to take your mind off smoking at all, in fact you want it to be rather more on smoking, and on how you're going about stopping doing it. Hiding from the reality of what you're doing is just another (slightly addictive) 'avoiding' response, and it doesn't work. One day you will come to, from your state of forgetfulness, to find yourself with a cigarette in hand, and realise that some nasty 'forgotten' need had come creeping up on you unawares and grabbed you from behind.

What I want to stress all along is that what you really need to get away from is the habit associated with smoking; in effect to take your body, rather than your mind, off smoking. And to do that you need to concentrate more, rather than less, on what you're doing. At the same time you want to focus on the replacement benefits you're picking up as you go, so that concentrating on what you're doing becomes a positive pleasure rather than a misery. When you're thinking, 'Win, win, win,' you will find that your mind will actually be able to deal with it all quite happily.

Thinking and living for success

We've spent quite a lot of time in this chapter looking at what smoking has been 'giving' us over the years, specifically in terms of the emotional and behavioural fulfilment we've told ourselves we've been getting. And we've also spent time considering what healthier alternatives to smoking we can come up with to deal with some of the significant needs we have. The second part, replacing what we've been conned into believing could help us with something more genuine, is vital because where there is a vacuum, nature will fill it rather than leave it empty. And we don't want to fill the space where smoking sat in our lives with something that will just have to be diarised forward as yet another problem. So far in this chapter I've made suggestions for alternative ways to fill each role that cigarette smoking has been playing in your life. They are ones that should act to reduce temptation in the short term, and to provide more fulfilment in the long term, but they are just that – suggestions. The best solutions will always be your own.

But as well as finding replacements for the individual emotional and behavioural satisfactions that we've had from cigarette smoking in the past, there is still more we can do to break our ties with smoking, and our need for cigarettes. We can do quite a bit to change the overall way we think and live.

I hope that doesn't sound either too surprising or too ambitious. For one thing, it was floated as an expectation at the start of the book. And for another, all the time you've been reading this book you've had it banged into your head that smoking isn't a single issue, that it belongs to a whole set of attitudes and behaviours that we have to revamp if we want to get over addiction completely. So why not tackle all of them at the same time and get the bonus of a healthier lifestyle, whilst getting over smoking?

The next part of this chapter will cover the straightforward things we can do, not only to make the stopping smoking process easier, but also to make a lot of other areas of our lives much more rewarding.

Getting more out of stopping smoking

The basic aim here is to make changes in lifestyle that bring overall benefits whilst also helping us avoid the situations most likely to 'trip' the sensory associations that there have been with our smoking past. It's similar to getting over an unhappy love affair, which is altogether easier if we consciously avoid the places and experiences that were shared with the unsatisfactory lover, and make efforts to get into a new (and better) relationship.

The following suggestions will be about creating either those changes in lifestyle or the background conditions that will make going about it all that little bit easier.

Helpful working conditions

Most of us find that we work better in comfortable conditions (what are we trying to prove if we don't?!), and the same goes for working through the process of stopping smoking and staying stopped. We want to feel comfortable while we're doing it. If we're not physically comfortable we are, as addictive types, more likely to feel resentful. And where does resentment take us? Back to 'neediness', demanding the comfort of a cigarette, of course. So, for the best possible chance of success, aim for comfort at all times:

- Keep warm. Feeling huddled and cold leaves us miserable, vulnerable, needy and also less able to make good judgments. You've got every reason (and the extra pennies, now) to keep your body temperature right.

- Wear clothes that make you feel good. We all have several wardrobes: one will be a 'comfy' wardrobe, another will be a 'smart' one and so on. Whilst you're going through the stopping smoking process, choose, as far as is practical, from the wardrobe labelled, 'really suits me and feels as comfortable as a second skin'. You want to build your morale and also develop a sense that as you're stopping smoking you're also making your personal space a lovelier one to be in.

- Spend money on getting your hair and teeth up to scratch – they've probably suffered from your smoking, anyway. Now, especially, you want to be able to enjoy the actual business of eating and to feel that your hair is behaving itself to the highest standards – and be as happy as you can with the feeling of being in your own body. Always keep hair and teeth as squeaky-clean as possible (and do your tongue as well – buy a scraper, or just brush it). You'll love them and yourself a whole lot more.

- If your hands and nails are in a mess, give them a make-over as well. Rid yourself of any reminders of nicotine and be pleased to look at your hands.

- If you've got other health problems, or just general aches and pains, go to your doctor and get them sorted as far as possible. Pain causes resentment and wears down resistance (if it didn't, there would be no torturers). You need to feel physically on top of things, or if not quite that, at least that you've got most of your physical problems covered, and you're not feeling too vulnerable.

- Surround yourself with pleasant stimuli – again, as far as is practical. Move your desk to access a prettier view; if your journey to work can be made more attractive by taking an alternative route, take it; bring colour or scent into your life by buying a picture or fresh flowers; and if you've got a pet at home, just stroke it a whole lot more.

Okay, you get the picture. It makes simple commercial sense. You've got a job to do. Look after yourself, and keep the worker happy.

Keep busy

Keeping busy in the early stages of stopping smoking will bring huge benefits. In the first place, being busy keeps us away from many of our old temptations and, in the second, being busy also brings its own solid rewards. We should quite simply (and fairly obviously) find that we get more done in a day, and we should also find that, almost by default, we set up a more efficient and morale-boosting routine for future living.

But merely keeping super-busy at work may possibly bring slightly negative effects. You may feel resentful if you find yourself taking on other people's work, or working twice as much as anyone else, and we know what that means. And you may be immersing yourself in the culture where you have smoked in the past anyway (see the sections on the culture of smoking in the workplace). Only go in for endless overtime if those negative possibilities don't apply.

Otherwise, to fill your evenings, you can get a tremendous sense of achievement, and even a perverse sense of adventure, from going through all those unvisited places in your home, like the backs of cupboards, the bottoms of drawers, or, if you're after the bigtime, the loft and the cellar. You never know what you're going to find, and, as all those TV lifestyle programmes point out, you'll feel that you're going through a healthful detox at the same time.

And there must be a million things you've been meaning to do for centuries, such as sending a lengthy e-mail to Aunt Sheila in Canberra, or mending the leaky tap in the shower room, or cross-referencing all your photos under both subject and year. If you achieve all these leftover tasks, you'll not only feel unbelievably pleased with yourself, you'll also set up new associations, between stopping smoking and a fantastically positive sense of achievement and self-respect.

New – and bad – addictive behaviour

People who are basically addictive in their thinking style don't do themselves any favours by becoming involved in new situations or behaviours that are as likely to turn addictive as the ones they're getting shot of. And that makes the question of exercise a little bit complicated. We've probably all heard of someone who has gone from being an overweight, chain-smoking workaholic or couch potato, to being a born-again, evangelical convert to the gym, triathlons and steroids. On page 105, I mentioned non-destructive ways of managing addiction to behaviour, and this is where they come in.

There's nothing wrong with doing things compulsively, as such. It's *what* we do compulsively that counts. Compulsive smoking rates pretty low on the scale of healthy compulsions. But compulsive exercising (especially when it comes with the use of extra hormones) is, perhaps surprisingly, not much better. Many an over-exerciser ends up suffering from bad health. On the other hand, a compulsive commitment to self-improvement, when the self-improvement comes with its own health checks included, has a lot of benefits going for it. So, if you must be addicted to a behaviour, be addicted to a form of behaviour that's going to help, rather than harm, you.

Exercise

Exercise is an absolutely brilliant way of retraining your brain and body to cope better. With the right amount of exercise you start to get a smarter, leaner look, which boosts your self-esteem; you get a more efficient system, which will demand more appropriate foodstuffs (and that makes it easier for you to turn off the sugars/fats/salts button); you clear the years of rubbish in your lungs and repair your blood pressure and cholesterol levels more quickly, too. Then, if you take your exercise in the fresh air, which is by far the best way, you get additional benefits from that. However, there is a level at which exercising may actually increase the temptations of addiction. For example – and this effect will vary from individual to individual – if you run for about two to three miles, you will start to produce endorphins, which are opiate-like chemicals that increase pleasure and reduce feelings of pain. The connection between such chemicals and addiction is pretty clear.

There are a number of ways of managing the potential for addiction that too much exercise can bring with it. One is to be aware of the danger and to make sure that you make your commitment to self-improvement, rather than to exercise itself. Another is to exercise in a social, but not overly competitive, setting, so that your friends can help you keep focused. If you're someone who absolutely must win at all costs, then you should probably avoid squash, and if you go to the gym, ask one of the professional trainers there to monitor the time you spend on equipment and the weights you use. Unless you mean to end up like Charles Atlas.

The moral is that for exercise to work for you it must be regulated and it must work to increase your self-respect, not your powers of self-absorption.

Diet

You can hardly turn the telly on today without hearing about the benefits of a sensible diet. A famous cartoon cat once said, 'You are what you eat, avoid fruits and nuts.' Which in its way is pretty good advice, only we don't mind being fruity, what we want to avoid is being fatty, chippy and addicted.

A lot of research suggests that brain disorders, behavioural problems and addiction are all made worse, if not actually sparked off, by a diet that is full of chemicals (found in processed foods and drinks), fats, sugars and salt. Wheat and dairy products are on the list of suspects, too. It seems that the more of all of these things we eat, the more we want. And, not only don't they satisfy, but they also leave us feeling either bloated, dull, achey and depressed, or hyper, neurotic, aggressive and depressed. Plus greedy for other types of toxins.

The trouble is that if we try to give up everything we've ever thought we enjoyed eating, on the off-chance that it's also been making us depressed and addictive, we're likely to feel so depressed about having to do it that we'll feel we need a fag to get over the depression. So, rather than ban all the goodies from our diet, we should go for sensible, achievable ways of improving our systems.

The easy bit will be banning unnecessary chemicals from our diet. We banish the chemicals by getting rid of the processed foods. They're expensive in any case and processed foods are just the food manufacturers' way of hijacking our taste buds and holding them up to ransom. Let's demand them back. Buy only natural foodstuffs for a couple of weeks and you'll rediscover taste buds you'd forgotten all about. You'll also fall in love with eating again, feel loads fitter, save money and, of course, find it much, much easier to live without those other unwanted toxins – cigarettes.

For the rest, spend time browsing through the health and nutrition sections of bookshops before you try out other, more personalised, dietary improvements. You want to end up feeling enthusiastic about what you're eating, as well as physically healthier. So be sure that any dietary changes you make are ones that bring variety and excitement into your life. Putting healthy, vitamin-rich meals together should give you ritual and manual activity, as well as good nutrition, but doing it should also be sensual, stimulating and fun (just think of Nigella Lawson). Who needs fags?

Fun

Speaking of fun, it should always play a part in our lives, but it's even more essential to have fun times when we're also doing something we might feel apprehensive about, like stopping smoking. We need to feel we're getting more, not less, fun out of life – so that we can associate as many positive feelings as possible with the stopping process. And the great thing is that when fun no longer has to be fitted around that old bully, smoking, we've got more time for it, and more opportunities for fun will be available to us.

If we've always associated having fun with smoking, we've either limited ourselves to doing things in smoker-friendly places, or to feeling deprived half the time. And we will probably also have associated other smoker-friendly activities with the package we called 'having fun'. Meaning that if we now want to divorce having fun from having fags, we might have to ditch the other parts of the package, too, at least for a while.

For example, a karaoke night at the pub will involve singing, booze, fags, smoky atmosphere, snacks and friends. If karaoke has been your thing in the past, you will have bought into the total package, and it will have been all of those things put together that you'll have associated with having fun. Once you've separated out the fags, the rest of it won't feel the same any more. Something will always seem to be missing, and then we're back with the vacuum again, the one that nature wants to fill.

Rather than trying to remake old ways of having fun, but with bits missing, you'll be better off finding new ones. After all, without cigarettes tyrannising your life, you've got lots of new opportunities. You're going to be a lot healthier, which will open up new possibilities for having physical fun; and you're going to be feeling freer, now that you don't always have to be looking for ways and places to smoke, which will open up options as well. So why not go in for fresh and different activities? You may even find yourself enjoying them so much that your pub friends become jealous and want to join you.

But if the attractions of what's left of the old karaoke package are too strong to resist for ever, at least take a break from them until all the old associations with fags have had time to weaken. Meantime, if you still want to sing karaoke, try singing in a different environment from the pub. It doesn't even have to be an alcohol-free one, as long as you break enough other links to smoking. You could always buy a karaoke machine for home, get in some wine and invite your friends round; or you could set up karaoke evenings in the village hall and raise funds for charity. The karaoke machine in the pub doesn't have to be an excuse for smoking.

Whether or not karaoke has ever been part of your life you could also think about taking up any of the following, non-cigarette-dependent ways of having fun:

- Playing cards, playing an instrument, playing parts in plays.

- Going sailing, going mountain climbing, going ice skating, going line dancing.

- Riding horses, riding motor bikes, riding killer waves.

Make a break with your past and find fresh new ways of having fun that stir up no particular associations with fags. The more physical the fun you're having, the more new, non-cigarette-related rewards you will be giving yourself, and the easier it will be for you to stick to stopping smoking.

And, in the early days of stopping smoking, while you're trying to get as much fun as possible into your life, you should also avoid doing things you would rate as distinctly 'non-fun' (see Resentment, page 123). Unless, of course, you think that taking your mother-in-law on a day trip to an out-of-town shopping centre is likely to give you such a sense of moral superiority it will keep your resolve going strong rather than sap your will to live.

The benefits

If you follow, more or less, the direction that this chapter is pointing you in, you'll not only find it easier to stick to what you're doing, but you'll also find it a lot more fulfilling. Stopping smoking should be thought of as *adding* something of real value to your life, and definitely not as *depriving* you of something that once had value. And the best way to put that positive spin on to stopping smoking is to fill any gaps that are left where smoking was taken out of your life, with healthier, more active and much more exciting alternatives.

Positive reinforcement

It will also be enormously helpful to talk absolutely positively to everyone about what you're doing. If you think and talk in a depressed way, and say things like, 'Oh, God! I've just got to stop smoking, but it's going to be murder,' you'll be surrounding yourself and your actions with negativity. To keep your morale high, talk yourself up, and let everyone know that this stopping smoking business is a positive step that you've chosen to take, and that you're immensely proud of what you're doing. In other words, *believe in yourself.* Remember these three things:

- You're in the process of discovering a brand new world.

- You're a pioneer.

- You're making yourself a new life.

And on the subject of other people, we all have two kinds of friends: those who support us and those who don't. For the time being at least, dump anyone who doesn't, for whatever reason, give you their full support as you're stopping smoking. And if they offer you a cigarette, again for whatever reason, what kind of friend are they?

Stopping smoking isn't about giving anything up, it's about adding things to your life. Apart from all the obvious and vital things that it's adding, like good health that might make your future life worth living, it's adding something that can hardly be overestimated in terms of the value it will add to your life. And that's the ability to cope on your own with all life can throw at you. When you stop smoking and learn to deal with life on its terms, you also give up addiction and become self-sufficient. It isn't only 1970s-style commune dwellers who can benefit from self-sufficiency. Being self-sufficient frees up your powers of thought, your concentration and your capacity to deal with problems all by yourself.

You've got an exciting new life ahead.

And because you want to live that life *free of the fear* of relapse, a fear that is as much of a life sentence as smoking can be itself, we're going to take a look at the ways you can deal with any possibility of temptation in the next chapter. It's here as much to create a sense of security as for any other reason. You shouldn't, and probably won't, need it. But it's always nice to know there's a safety net when you're taking new steps into the future.

Relapse Prevention
Or, No going back

We don't want to contemplate relapse. We don't want to contemplate failure. And quite right, too. We want only positive thoughts about stopping smoking, and that's why this chapter is here. When we get to the end of a, 'How to become absolutely everything you've ever dreamed of being' style of book, we feel all confident and 'up'. We feel we can do it, yes sir! And that's exactly how we need to feel so that we've got the drive to ensure everything works for us. But at the same time we still need to be realists and to know something about what we might have to deal with once that first upbeat period is over.

It's much the same thing as when I said that we shouldn't be trying to forget about cigarettes as we're stopping smoking, we should only be trying to break the links we have had with them. If we try to make something go away simply by pretending it isn't there any longer, it won't work. That way it's much more likely to take us by surprise than if we acknowledge its existence. We need to realise that it still retains the potential to control us, and so take steps to protect ourselves against it. It's not at all the same thing as being frightened of it, nor is it the same as contemplating relapse and failure. It's thinking about potential causes of them, and making plans to protect ourselves against them. In fact, it's very positive thinking.

So, the great thing to focus on is, we've made it! You've stopped smoking, and you're feeling really good about yourself. Relapse isn't going to happen, because you're going to be ready for it. You're going to be protected against it. And this is the way it's going to work.

Handling crisis times

Once the euphoria of stopping smoking has worn off a bit, you'll find yourself becoming slightly blasé, rather used to the idea that you're a non-smoker. Which is wonderful, as long as you also remember that you were *originally* a non-smoker, before you started smoking in the first place. Your current non-smoker status will last as long as you keep the original gremlins – the ones that got you smoking in the first place – in mind, and at bay. In other words, as long as you remember everything that you have read in this book.

You're bound to have 'down times' in the future, and though they may not be directly related to stopping smoking, when they happen you should still remember all that you have covered during this stopping smoking process. And you must use all your new skills to deal with any down times and crises, otherwise if you think, 'This is nothing to do with stopping smoking,' and go back to your old ways you will find temptation tapping you on the shoulder and whispering in your ear. And this is what it will sound like:

'Oh, sod it. I don't really feel I *need* cigarettes any longer, so surely I can afford to have an occasional one. Especially when I'm under such pressure. It won't do any harm and I won't go back to smoking once this little spot of bother is over. I'll be fine again.'

Or it might come dressed up as autopilot. You'll just be cruising along through those challenging times (and challenge can be about excitement, as well as about depression – remember?). And lo and behold – there you are, with a fag in hand! How on earth did that happen?

Crisis times, almost by definition, push all those old emotional buttons of ours, and so default reactions like those just mentioned become very likely. In the Army, they understand the psychology behind all of this as well as anyone. Which is why the Army trains its soldiers so very, very hard. An army has to be able to depend on its soldiers' reactions and so they hyper-train them until they've replaced any unwanted default reactions with totally useful new ones.

And so that you can have the same strengths that they have in the Army, and the security of knowing that you're able to depend on your own reactions in times of crisis, you're going to follow their lead. Don't, whatever else you do, leave this next bit of advice out. It will really benefit you.

Go back to the critical moment of choice

You have to do this *straight away,* at this point in your reading. Go back to the chapter entitled, Going Critical, starting on page 86, and reread it. And don't cheat by side-stepping it, because you'll only be cheating yourself.

You need to be as familiar with the whole of the process covered in that chapter as the back of your hand. Revisit the chapter regularly. You want the whole history of how you used to get to the point of grabbing for a fag, of how you used to get to the critical moment of choice, etched on your memory. And then you need to train yourself very, very hard to make sure that your default route away from the critical moment remains Route Two, the one where you don't light up.

Make a list of likely crisis times

Having reminded yourself of what used to be needed to get you smoking, the next thing you should do is make a list of what you imagine could be potential times when those old thought-patterns and feelings might come up again. For example, if you've decided that a critical moment of choice often came after you'd had a bad day at work (when you were left feeling out of control and inadequate), that would suggest three separate situations in which you might remain more vulnerable to temptation than usual:

- A bad day at work (surprise, surprise!).

- Situations where others are in charge and you feel you could lose control over your life.

- Situations that result in you feeling inadequate.

Maybe it sounds too obvious or just very 'picky', but it always helps to actually put down in words what you think you internally 'know' (without having to say it). It makes it easier then to ask yourself direct questions about what's going on inside. For example, 'I'm having a bad day at work. So how do I really feel about it, and should I be on my guard against the possibility of a "critical moment"'? Asking yourself a direct question in that simple a way will be really helpful and positive.

So, make that list. Forewarned is forearmed.

Develop a positive attitude to crisis situations

Once you can predict likely crisis situations, you're in the position of being able to take control over what happens next. All you then need, in order to deal calmly and positively with any temptation you might feel, is to be sure that your basic attitude to crises is as helpful as possible.

This isn't the place to examine whether what might be happening to you is a real or an imagined crisis. We covered that sort of question earlier on, when we were looking at addictive thinking. What we're talking about here is whether you see crisis times as positive or negative.

And though your attitude will relate back to the coping mechanisms and attitudes you developed as a child, we need to deal with it as a separate issue here, because it's very much involved in relapse prevention.

Where are you when it comes to a crisis: on the side of the negatives, or the positives?

Negative thinking

- Do you see a crisis as a setback? As something that will set challenges you can't cope with and inevitably lead to a sense of despair?

- In the event of a momentary failure to stick to something you've undertaken, do you think, 'Oh, heck, here we go again'?

- Do you feel you recognise where you are when you fail at something, that you feel like you're on home territory?

- Do you see a crisis as inevitably having a negative outcome, as something bad?

- If you're getting something wrong, do you feel, 'Might as well be hung for a sheep as a lamb'? And see no point in trying to minimise the damage?

- When faced with a challenge, do you fear failure too much to expose yourself to any risk?

If the answer to any of those questions is 'Yes', then you have what is basically a negative attitude to challenge and crisis times.

Positive thinking

In order to deal with temptation better, you need to work on developing more of the following positive style of thinking.

- When you feel a crisis coming on, think, 'This is just the time to test out my coping skills. I want to prove to myself that I can do it.'

- In the event of failure, think, 'Oh, bugger, I'd better see what I can do to get something out of this situation. In any case, it's not the end of the world.'

- Start finding out what success feels like and learn how to live with it naturally.

- Think: 'Nothing ventured, nothing gained'.

- When things are going wrong, try to minimise the damage, and don't feel you're stuck with viewing a short-term failure to get things right as a long-term disaster.

- Remember: 'I'll risk failure because I'm going all out for success'.

If you keep repeating positive thoughts like these instead of the negative thoughts in the first list, you'll be training yourself to deal with crisis times in an upbeat way. If crises come you'll be able to say 'No' to negativity and 'No' to temptation. And that means you'll stay away from smoking.

And the end result with positive thinking can be even better than that, because going through a crisis can then actually bring you benefits. If you use positive, rather than negative, thoughts to talk yourself through a critical situation, your levels of self-knowledge and self-respect will grow enormously. Positive is as positive does.

Should you actually have a 'blip' and decide to smoke a cigarette, or even two, the way you think about what you've done is still all-important. I'm not suggesting that having that cigarette would actually be a positive thing, or that you should see it as insignificant, but one failure needn't mean that you have to give up in despair. As long as you think about the 'blip' in a positive way, you can keep it as a one-off lapse, rather than allowing it to knock you off course. You don't have to be stuck with thinking, 'That's it, I'm a smoker again.'

Instead, as I recommended earlier, revisit Going Critical, and go through the chapter quickly. Take the attitude that you're just having to reset your new default mode because it had a little hiccup. And with positive thinking that's all it need amount to.

Remember you always have access to your two-part relapse prevention strategy:

- Keep reminding yourself of how you came to take up smoking, and of how you now have the choice of a better option, by frequently revisiting Going Critical. Each visit is a form of training reinforcement.

- Use only positive thinking about your ability to cope.

If you keep doing those two things, you may have no need to use them as a strategy for dealing with relapse. They'll be acting as your *relapse prevention* tools.

More helpful hints

These are a few, last-minute, extra resources, which you can turn to for support and 'topping up' whenever they might be helpful. Use them if they are helpful. Ignore them if they're not.

If you're having problems with trigger feelings (see page 46) practise diversionary tactics. Treat a trigger feeling as if it were a toddler having a tantrum – which in effect it is – and divert it. Take it for a walk, literally, both to change the scenery and to use up some of its energy. Amuse it, make it laugh; laughter is a brilliant way of changing brain chemistry anyway, so your feelings are bound to change when you laugh. To amuse yourself, think of Basil Fawlty, or keep in mind a ready supply of funny things that have happened to you. And you could always get someone to tickle you!

Try a homeopathic approach to symptom reduction. If you feel anger, let some out a bit at a time in a non-destructive way; by punching a punchball, for instance. You'll feel it being satisfied without causing harm. If you feel constant anxiety, let some out in a non-neurotic way; why not feel concerned with the health of the nation, say. You'll feel your anxiety's being validated without having to rip yourself to shreds.

Imagine that your long-held, but outdated, attitudes are like items of comfortable clothing that you've worn into holes. Try out some smarter new looks from time to time and you'll feel quite differently about yourself. For example, if your attitude has always been, 'I should be in control,' slip into, 'I should find life stimulating,' instead. You'll be amazed at the effect. Like changing from DIY overalls into a designer suit, you suddenly realise how differently you're walking and talking. So prepare yourself for a makeover.

Play around with the way you say things to yourself. Standard cause and effect thinking (such as, 'If I smoke when I'm young, then I will have health problems when I'm older') doesn't work for everyone. Try out some variations on ways of saying that to yourself, for example, 'When I have a cigarette I'm hurting myself inside.' Or, 'I can have a cigarette and feel a bit good for now, or on the other hand I could refuse a cigarette now and feel much better soon.'

If you come across problems as you're taking the stopping smoking path, imagine that they're like ditches on your way to where you're going. Do you stop, then turn back when you come to them, or do you quickly leap over them and get on with your journey?

- Practise delaying tactics. It's a skill we could all do with practising in the modern world. So when you want a cup of coffee, make do with a glass of water (to quench your thirst) for a while. Wait for a good 30 minutes before you have the coffee, you'll enjoy it all the more. When you want a treat, such as a piece of chocolate, finish some necessary task before you have it. And then when you do have it, concentrate on eating it, and don't work or read at the same time. Psychologists all agree that delaying gratification leads to greater satisfaction and better coping skills.

- Practise getting some positive results into each day of your life. Set yourself at least one smallish, achievable goal every day – for example, taking five minutes exercise, reading a chapter of a book you've always meant to read, or repairing or polishing something. It's amazing how good you'll feel to know you've done it.

- Practise breathing. Most people don't breathe properly, and smokers are the worst of all. Deep breathing, down to the tummy, helps calm the mind and settle the body. It needs to be practised. But it's invaluable in a crisis.

- Drink lots of still water and green tea. Both cleanse the system and help you feel pure – you'll want to stay that way.

- Create a positive mantra for yourself and quietly chant it to yourself on a regular basis. 'Every day, in every way, I'm getting better and better,' worked wonders for people in the early part of the twentieth century. Perhaps you could use something like, 'I needn't be needy', or, 'It's never too big to deal with,' or how about, 'Good health, great wealth.' It really is your choice.

The Sweet Smell of Success

Or, Congratulations, you've given up

Congratulations, *congratulations, CONGRATULATIONS!*

You've worked very hard so you deserve absolutely everything that you've achieved.

And haven't you got so much more out of reading this book than you ever bargained for when you bought it? Apart from the holy grail of stopping smoking, you've also come away with ideas that will change the way you see things for the rest of your life. You've had to face some pretty tough challenges to the way you think as you've been reading, and by coming through it all you've shown open-mindedness, sticking power and courage. And now you've finished the course with flying colours, so give yourself a great big hug and a pat on the back.

Then there's the goodie bag that you've got to take away with you as well. If you remember, it carries the promise of changes in your life, your finances, and your relationships once you've reached the end of the book. And that's in addition to stopping smoking.

You get those extras because, unlike other quitting smoking techniques, which tackle smoking as a single issue, this book has helped you to see that smoking behaviour is part of a much bigger picture and is only one of a range of other, similar, behaviours. And that as you challenge the *underlying* causes of any one of these behaviours, you will inevitably make changes in all the others.

You've had to learn a lot about yourself as you've been looking for those underlying causes of your behaviour, and that has turned you into a slightly different person from the one who first picked up this book. You've been growing and developing as you've been reading, and now you should be able to understand yourself and the motivations that have driven your behaviour better than you've ever done before. And that will inevitably lead to improvements in your life and relationships. As for the financial benefits you're getting from stopping smoking, and from avoiding other addictions, they should speak for themselves.

From the start you've had to do quite radical things.

- You had to *take responsibility for your own behaviour.* You had to kill the 'smoking monster'; the idea that smoking was a 'thing' that had power over you. You had to accept responsibility for the series of actions that you were carrying out each time you smoked, and you had to recognise that you had a choice in whether or not you did those things.

- You had to *see yourself as others see you,* and stop making excuses for yourself. By looking at what you were doing from the outside in, you could start to be more honest with yourself about your smoking behaviour. You could think more objectively about what might lie behind it; and you could treat yourself to the very sensible advice (and genuine understanding) that a truly sympathetic onlooker should be able to give you.

Once you could start to move away from the almost instinctive denials of the past, and could think more objectively about what might lie behind your smoking behaviour, you embarked on a new, quite complicated process. You began to work out how you developed an addictive neediness that demanded the chemical rush and the rituals of cigarettes simply for you to be able to manage your feelings.

And you came to recognise that:

- Smoking is not a monster which lives outside ourselves, but is an *inner* need for chemicals which will 'help' us to manage our needy feelings.

- Smoking is not a monster that lives outside us, but is a sequence of silly *behaviours of our own,* which we always have the capacity to control.

- Smoking, as such, doesn't really exist. We perform series of ritual actions with chemical-producing objects we call cigarettes, but the notion that this all amounts to something in its own right which has the ability to bring anything of genuine value into our lives, really is *all in the mind.*

And that means that it really is only in the mind that we can give smoking up.

You saw that every smoker regularly arrives at critical moments of choice, programmed by the past, when a decision has to be taken about whether or not to set light to a cigarette. Nobody forces that decision, it's the smoker's mind alone that decides what their body is going to do next. Just for that one second, we always have the choice, the absolute potential to be or not to be a smoker.

In order that you could see the whole of that truth as clearly as possible, you made yourself a splendid wall chart. On it you showed everything, mental, emotional, psychological and historical, that had gone into the making of you and your 'critical moment of choice'. And next to that you showed where you would be going if you took the decision to light up at that moment, and where you would be going if you took the decision *not* to light up at that moment.

You could see, perhaps for the very first time, that the choice of behaviour you have been making in the past (to light up) had too much to do with you actually being stuck in the past. For a more independent future, your mind would have to be set free to make the choice that would be good for you.

And from the chart you could also see just how simple it is to become a non-smoker, for good. With all the benefits that brings in terms of lifestyle, health and wealth.

You've completed the process now and perhaps it feels as though you've lived a miniature lifetime since you started reading. Which would be a perfectly natural thing to feel, because as you've been reading you have actually been reborn, both as a non-smoker, and as someone who can cope better with life generally. With the help of this book you've not only discovered how to stop smoking, you've also learned how to avoid falling for any alternative forms of addiction. You're a new independent.

So welcome to a new world. You're a pioneer in this new world of yours. And you've got a whole new life ahead of you – it's yours to make of it what you want.

You're in a win-win-win situation, because:

- You've stopped setting light to cigarettes.

- You've given up addictive thinking, chemical overload, instant gratification and smokescreens.

And, best of all,

- You've taken up control of your life.

CONGRATULATIONS!

Index